Cardiology Words and Phrases

A Quick-Reference Guide

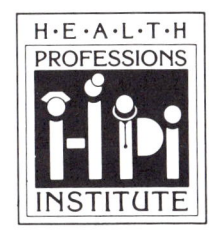

Health Professions Institute • Modesto, California • 1989

Cardiology Words and Phrases:
A Quick-Reference Guide

© 1989, Health Professions Institute.
All rights reserved.

Developed by:
Health Professions Institute
801 15th Street, Suite E
Modesto, California 95354
Telephone (209) 524-4351

Published by:

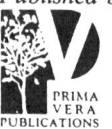

Prima Vera Publications
P. O. Box 801
Modesto, California 95353
Telephone (209) 524-4351
Sally C. Pitman, Editor & Publisher

Printed by:
Parks Printing & Lithograph
Modesto, California

ISBN 0-934385-16-5

Last digit is the print number: 9 8 7 6 5 4 3

Preface

The primary source for **Cardiology Words and Phrases** is *The SUM Program Cardiology Transcription Unit* (1989). These educational materials are part of The SUM (**S**ystems **U**nit **M**ethod) Program for training medical transcriptionists, developed by Health Professions Institute.

Numerous transcripts of cardiology medical and surgical dictation, as well as textbooks, scholarly journals, and other references, were carefully reviewed to select more than 15,000 cardiology words and phrases. The resulting quick-reference guide is a useful reference to medical transcriptionists and other health-care professionals who encounter cardiology terminology. A list of selected references begins on page 185.

Many medical transcriptionists and other health-care professionals contributed to this effort by providing word lists or reviewing transcripts: Nancy Barker, CMT, Modesto, Ca.; Charlotte R. Bowers, RRA, Baltimore, Md.; Jenola Bradwell, CMT, ART, Orlando, Fl.; Patricia A. Collins, CMT, Mission Viejo, Ca.; Genevieve Dean, RN, Daly City, Ca.; Beverly S. Hunter, CMT, Orlando, Fl.; Norma Lopresti, CMT, Bethlehem, Pa.; Norene Schillaci, Daly City, Ca.; Bron Taylor, CMT, San Francisco, Ca.; Donna M. Taylor, CMT, Santa Ana, Ca.; Susan Verdier, CMT, Orlando, Fl.; Linda Vourlogianes, Petaluma, Ca; and Kathleen Mors Woods, Baltimore, Md.

This reference book was produced by the staff and associates of Health Professions Institute: Susan M. Turley, CMT, RN, Curriculum Coordinator, Baltimore; Linda C. Campbell, CMT, Educational Coordinator, Modesto; Vera Pyle, CMT, Consulting Editor, San Francisco; and John H. Dirckx, M.D., Medical Consultant, Dayton, Ohio.

Our warmest gratitude to all.

Sally C. Pitman, CMT, MA
Editor & Publisher

How To Use This Book

The cardiology words and phrases in this reference are listed alphabetically and are extensively cross-referenced. An eponymic title may be located alphabetically as well as under the term that it modifies. For example, *Siemens-Pacesetter pacemaker* may be found under both *Siemens-Pacesetter* and the main entry *pacemaker*. Eponyms are not presented in the possessive form ('s), although they are frequently used as possessives in medical reports and literature.

Selected medications used frequently in cardiology and cardiac surgery are located only under the main entry *medication*— not alphabetically throughout the book.

To minimize unnecessary duplications, many subentries are combined under one main entry. The main entry *operation* includes all cardiac surgical procedures, which are also found alphabetically throughout the book under their respective titles.

A few main entries with multiple subentries are listed below.

anastomosis	heart	retractor
aneurysm	hypertension	rhythm
angina	infarction	risk factors
artery	interval	scissors
block	lead	shunt
bypass	leaflet	sign
cannula	medication	sound
catheter	murmur	stenosis
clamp	myocarditis	suture
contrast medium	operation	syndrome
defect	pacemaker	system
disease	pacing	tachycardia
echocardiogram	pericarditis	technique
electrocardiogram	period	test
electrode	pressure	time
endocarditis	prosthesis	tube
forceps	protocol	valve
gradient	pulse	volume
graft	rate	wall
guide wire	ratio	wave

Cardiology Words and Phrases

A

"a" (augment)(ed)
"a" dip on echocardiogram
"a" wave of jugular venous pulse
  Cannon
  giant
A fib (atrial fibrillation) pattern
A-line (arterial)
A-mode echocardiography
A point
A wave of cardiac apex pulse
A wave pressure on atrial catheterization
AA (ascending aorta)
AA curve; A_1A_2 curve
AA interval; A_1A_2 interval
A_2 equal to P_2; A_2 greater than P_2
A_2 heart sound (aortic valve closure)
A_2 incisural interval
A_2/MVO interval (aortic valve closure/mitral valve opening)
AAA (abdominal aortic aneurysm)
AACD (abdominal aortic counterpulsation device)
AAI (atrial demand inhibited) pacemaker
AAI rate-responsive mode
AAT (atrial demand triggered) pacemaker
ABE (acute bacterial endocarditis)
aberrant conduction
aberrant coronary artery
aberrant QRS complex
aberrantly conducted beats
aberration, nonspecific T wave
ABG (arterial blood gas) (see *blood gas*)

ABI (ankle-brachial index)
ablation
  accessory conduction (ACA)
  atrioventricular nodal
  electrode catheter
  endocardial catheter
  His bundle
  Kent bundle
  transcatheter His bundle
  transcoronary chemical
  transvenous
ablation of pathway, surgical
abnormality
  akinetic wall motion
  baseline ST segment
  brisk wall motion
  exercise-induced wall motion
  LV (left ventricular) wall motion
  nonspecific T wave
  perfusion
  persistent wall motion
  regional wall motion
  transient wall motion
  wall motion
abscess, aortic root
absolute cardiac dullness (ACD)
absolute refractory period (ARP)
AC (aortic closure) interval
ACA (accessory conduction ablation)
accelerator globulin (AcG) blood coagulation factor
accessory pathway
accident, cerebrovascular (CVA)
Accucap CO_2/O_2 monitor
Accu-Chek

1

Accucom cardiac output monitor
Accufix pacemaker lead
Acculith pacemaker
Accutorr monitor
ACE (angiotensin converting enzyme) inhibitor
ACE (asymptomatic complex ectopy)
ace of spades sign on angiogram
ACG (apex cardiogram)
AcG (accelerator globulin) blood coagulation factor
acid phosphatase
ACLS (advanced cardiac life support) protocol
acoustic window
acquired ventricular septal defect (AVSD)
acrocyanosis
ACS (Advanced Catheter Systems; Cardiovascular Systems)
ACS angioplasty Y connector
ACS guide wire
ACS Indeflator
ACS JL4 (Judkins left 4 French) catheter
ACS LIMA guide
ACS Mini catheter
ACS RX coronary dilatation catheter
ACS SULP II balloon
action potential
action potential duration (APD)
activated partial thromboplastin time (APTT)
active fixation lead
Activitrax variable rate pacemaker
acute bacterial endocarditis (ABE)
acute myocardial infarction (AMI)
AD (aortic diameter)
Adams-Stokes disease; syndrome
Adams-Stokes syncope
adapter
 butterfly
 side-arm
 sleeve
adherent pericardium
adhesion(s)
 freeing up of
 pericardial
 taking down of
ad hoc
Adolph's Salt Substitute
adrenergic drive; receptor
Adriamycin cardiotoxicity
Adson forceps; hook; maneuver; test
advanced cardiac life support (ACLS)
adventitious heart sounds
AECG (ambulatory ECG)
AED (automatic external defibrillator)
Ae-H interval
AEI (atrial escape interval)
Aequitron pacemaker
Aerobicycle (powered treadmill)
Aerodyne bicycle
AET (automatic ectopic tachycardia)
AF (atrial fibrillation; aortic flow; atrial flutter)
AFBG (aortofemoral bypass graft)
AFl (atrial flutter)
AFP pacemaker
afterload, cardiac
afterload reduction
AG (anion gap)
agglutinins, febrile
agonal tracing (on EKG)
AH curve; interval
AHA (American Heart Association)
AHC (apical hypertrophic cardiomyopathy)
AH:HA ratio
AHT (arterial hypertension)
AI (aortic insufficiency)
AICA (anterior inferior communicating artery)
AICD (automatic implantable or internal cardioverter defibrillator)

AICD-B and AICD-BR cardioverter defibrillator
AICD pacemaker
AICD shocks
AID (automatic implantable defibrillator)
AID-B defibrillator; pacemaker
airway, esophageal obturator
AK (atrial kick)
akinesia, akinesis, akinetic
akinesia, regional
akinesis, apical
akinetic left ventricle
akinetic posterior wall
Akutsu total artificial heart
albumin solution
Albuminar-5; -25
Albutein
Alcock catheter plug
Alexander rib raspatory
Alexander rib stripper
Alexander-Faraheuf rib rasp
Alfred M. Large vena cava clamp
algorithm
aliasing (in Doppler studies)
aliquot dose
alkaline phosphatase
alkalosis
Allen test prior to radial artery cannulation
Allen-Brown criteria
alligator pacing cable
Allis forceps
Allison lung retractor
allograft, cryopreserved human aortic
ALMD (asymptomatic left main disease)
Aloka echocardiograph machine
alpha$_1$-adrenergic blocker agent
alpha receptor
alternans
  electrical
  pulsus
  total

ALVAD (abdominal left ventricular assist device)
AMA-Fab (antimyosin monoclonal antibody with Fab fragment)
AMA-Fab scintigraphy
amaurosis fugax
Amberlite particles
AMC needle
American Heart Association (AHA) classification of stenosis
American Optical oximeter
AMI (acute or anterior myocardial infarction)
Amipaque contrast medium
AML (anterior mitral leaflet)
A-mode echocardiography
amp (amplitude)
Amplatz cardiac catheter
Amplatz dilator
Amplatz femoral catheter
Amplatz right coronary catheter
Amplatz Super Stiff guide wire
Amplatz torque wire
amplitude
  aortic
  apical IVS
  C-A mitral valve
  cardiac signal
  D-E
  diminished wave
  low
  mid-IVS
  posterior LV wall
  R wave
  septal
  valve opening
amplitude of EKG wave
amplitude of motion
amplitude of pulse
amplitude of QRS complex
amyloid, cardiac
amyloidosis
  senile cardiac
  systemic
ANA (antinuclear antibody) test

anacrotic limb of carotid arterial
    pulse
anacrotic notch of carotid arterial
    pulse
analysis, arterial blood gas
anasarca
anastomosis
  aorticopulmonary
  ascending aorta to pulmonary
      artery
  Baffe
  bidirectional cavopulmonary
  Blalock-Taussig
  cavopulmonary
  cobra-head
  Cooley intrapericardial
  Cooley modification of
      Waterston
  end-to-end
  end-to-side
  Glenn
  internal mammary artery to
      coronary artery
  Kugel
  left pulmonary artery to
      descending aorta
  portosystemic
  Potts
  Potts-Smith side-to-side
  precapillary
  right atrium to pulmonary artery
  right pulmonary artery to
      ascending aorta
  right subclavian to pulmonary
      artery
  side-to-side
  Sucquet-Hoyer
  superior vena cava to distal right
      pulmonary artery
  superior vena cava to pulmonary
      artery
  systemic to pulmonary artery
  tensionless
  Waterston extrapericardial
anastomosis arteriolovenularis
anastomosis arteriovenosa
anastomosis of Riolan
anastomotic
anatomy
  distorted
  left-dominant coronary
  right-dominant coronary
anchor, anchored
Anderson-Keys method for total
    serum cholesterol
Andrews suction tip
Andrews Pynchon suction tube
Anel method
anemia, anemic
anesthesia, crash induction of
aneurysm
  abdominal aortic (AAA)
  ampullary
  aortic
  aortoiliac
  arterial
  arteriosclerotic
  arteriovenous
  atherosclerotic
  axillary
  berry
  brain
  cardiac
  cerebral
  Charcot-Bouchard
  cirsoid
  compound
  coronary artery
  Crawford technique for
  cylindroid
  DeBakey technique for
  descending thoracic
  dissecting
  ectatic
  embolic
  false
  fusiform
  hernial
  infected
  innominate

aneurysm *(cont.)*
  intracranial
  lateral
  left ventricular
  mesh-wrapping of aortic
  miliary
  mixed
  mural
  mycotic
  orbital
  Park
  pelvic
  Potts
  racemose
  Rasmussen
  renal
  Richet
  Rodriguez
  ruptured atherosclerotic
  sacciform
  saccular; sacculated
  serpentine
  Shekelton
  sinus of Valsalva
  spindle-shaped
  spurious
  suprasellar
  syphilitic
  thoracic
  thoracoabdominal
  traumatic
  true
  tubular
  varicose
  venous
  ventricular
  verminous
  windsock
  worm
  wrapping of abdominal aortic
aneurysm cavity
aneurysm of sinus of Valsalva
aneurysmal bruit
aneurysmal bulging
aneurysmal dilatation
aneurysmal wall
aneurysmectomy, apicoseptal
aneurysmoplasty, Matas
ANF (atrial natriuretic factor)
Angell-Shiley bioprosthetic valve
Angell-Shiley xenograft prosthetic valve
Anger-type scintillation camera
angina (angina pectoris)
  accelerated
  atypical
  bandlike
  chronic stable
  classic
  clinical
  cold-induced
  coronary spastic
  coronary vasospastic
  crescendo
  crescendo-decrescendo
  eating-induced
  effort
  esophageal
  excruciatingly painful
  exercise-induced
  exertional
  focal
  gradual onset of
  Heberden
  intractable
  new onset
  nocturnal
  pacing-induced
  post-AMI
  postinfarction
  postprandial
  preinfarction
  Prinzmetal variant
  progressive
  recurrent
  refractory
  rest
  retrosternal heaviness with
  stable
  sudden onset of

angina *(cont.)*
    treadmill-induced
    typical effort
    unstable
    variable threshold
    variant
    vasomotor
    vasospastic
    vasotonic
    walk-through
angina, descriptions of:
    brought on or precipitated by
        anxiety
        cold weather
        eating a heavy meal
        emotional stress; upset
        exercise
        exertion
        exposure to cold
        heavy meals
        sexual intercourse
        smoking
        straining at the stool
        stress
        worry/anxiety
    burning feeling
    crushing chest pain
    elephant on chest feeling
    feeling of impending doom
    gradual onset
    heartburn-type feeling
    heaviness in chest
    indigestion-like feeling
    pinching chest pain
    precordial chest pain
    pressure-like sensation
    radiating down/into
        arm
        epigastrium
        fingers
        jaw
        left arm
        left shoulder
        neck
        scapula

angina *(cont.)*
    referred chest pain
    retrosternal burning; heaviness
    smothering sensation
    squeezing chest discomfort
    substernal burning
    sudden onset
    suffocating chest pain
    tightness of chest
angina after meals
angina at low work load
angina at rest
angina cordis
angina cruris
angina decubitus
angina inversa
angina of first effort
angina pectoris (see *angina*)
angina provoked by ergonovine
    maleate
angina unrelieved by nitroglycerin
angina vasomotoria
anginal equivalent
angiocardiography (see *angiogram*)
Angiocath
angiocatheter
    Deseret
    Eppendorf
    Mikro-tip
Angio-Conray contrast medium
Angiocor prosthetic valve
angiodysplasia
angiodysplastic lesion
angioedema
angiogram (angiocardiogram)
    biplane orthogonal
    Brown-Dodge method for
    cardiac
    cerebral
    cine
    contrast
    coronary
    digital subtraction (DSA)
    ECG-synchronized digital sub-
        traction

angiogram *(cont.)*
  equilibrium radionuclide
  first-pass nuclide rest and
    exercise
  first-pass radionuclide
  fluorescein
  gated blood pool
  gated nuclear
  gated radionuclide
  left ventricular
  post angioplasty
  PTCA coronary
  pulmonary
  pulmonary artery wedge
  radionuclide (RNA)
  rest and exercise gated nuclear
  selective coronary cine
  single plane
  sitting-up view
  transvenous digital subtraction
  ventricular
angiogram suite
angiographically
angiohemophilia
Angio-Kit catheter
angioplasty
  balloon
  coronary artery
  Dotter-Judkins technique for percutaneous transluminal
  Gruentzig balloon catheter
  laser
  multilesion
  one-vessel
  patch
  patch-graft
  percutaneous laser
  percutaneous transluminal (PTA)
  percutaneous transluminal coronary (PTCA)
  peripheral laser (PLA)
  supported
  transluminal
  transluminal balloon
  transluminal coronary artery

angioreticuloendothelioma of heart
angiosarcoma of heart
angioscope
  Mitsubishi
  Olympus
angiotensin converting enzyme (ACE) inhibitor
Angiovist contrast medium
angle
  cardiodiaphragmatic
  cardiohepatic
  cardiophrenic
  Ebstein
  nail-to-nailbed (clubbing)
  phase
  phrenopericardial
  Pirogoff
  QRS-T
  venous
angle of the jaw, jugular venous distention to the
Angled Balloon catheter
anion gap (AG)
anisoylated plasminogen streptokinase activator complex (APSAC)
Ankeney chest (sternal) retractor
ankle-arm index
ankle-brachial index (ABI)
annular abscess
annular calcification
annular constriction
annular dilatation
annular disruption
annular fracture
annular plication
annuli fibrosi cordis
annulocuspid hinge
annuloplasty (preferred over anuloplasty)
annuloplasty
  Carpentier
  De Vega
  prosthetic ring
  septal

annuloplasty *(cont.)*
   tricuspid valve
  annulus (or anulus)
   aortic valve
   calcified
   friable
   mitral
   pulmonary
   septal tricuspid
   valve
  anode, transvenous
  anomalous conduction
  anomalous origin of coronary artery
  anomalous pulmonary venous return
  anomalous retroesophageal right subclavian artery
  anomaly
   aortic arch
   cardiac
   congenital cardiac
   conotruncal congenital
   Ebstein
   Shone
   Taussig-Bing
   Uhl
  anoxia, anoxic
  ANP (atrial natriuretic polypeptide)
  antagonist, beta
  antecubital approach for cardiac catheterization
  antecubital approach for catheter insertion
  antecubital fossa; space
  antegrade conduction
  antegrade fashion, catheter advanced in an
  antegrade flow
  antegrade refractory period
  anterior internodal pathway
  anterior motion of posterior mitral valve leaflet
  anterior table
  anterior view on thallium imaging
  anteroapical
  anterolateral
  anteroseptal myocardial infarction
  antiadrenergic agent
  antianginal agent; drug; therapy
  antiarrhythmia agent; drug
  antibiotic
   perioperative
   postoperative
   preoperative
  antibiotic solution
  antibiotics, prophylactic
  antibody
   antimyosin monoclonal (with Fab fragment) (AMA-Fab)
   antinuclear (ANA)
   anticardiolipin (aCL)
   indium-111 antimyosin
   polyclonal anticardiac myosin
   sheep antidigoxin Fab
   teichoic acid
  anticardiolipin (aCL) antibody (aCL)
  anticoagulant, oral
  anticoagulant therapy
  anticoagulation, long-term
  antidromic tachycardia
  antiembolic stockings
  antifibrin antibody imaging
  antihemophilic blood coagulation factor
  antihyperlipidemic drug
  antihypertensive drug; therapy
  antinuclear antibody (ANA)
  antitachycardia pacing
  antithrombin III
  Antyllus method
  anuloplasty (see *annuloplasty*)
  anulus, anular (see *annulus*)
  anxiolytic
  AO (aorta; aortic; aortic opening)
  AO/AC (aortic valve opening/aortic valve closing) ratio

aorta
  abdominal
  ascending (AA)
  biventricular origin of
  calcified
  central
  coarctation of
  cross-clamping of
  descending
  dextropositioned
  double-barreled
  dynamic
  infrarenal abdominal
  kinked
  overriding
  palpable
  porcelain
  preductal coarctation of
  terminal
  thoracic
aorta abdominalis
aorta ascendens
aorta sacrococcygea
aorta thoracica
aortic annulus
aortic arch syndrome
aortic bulb
aortic closure (AC)
aortic configuration of cardiac
  shadow on x-ray
aortic cusps' separation
aortic diameter (AD)
aortic incompetency
aortic insufficiency (AI)
aortic opening (AO)
aortic override
aortic pullback
aortic regurgitation (AR)
aortic root perfusion needle
aortic root ratio
aortic stenosis (AS)
aortic thromboembolism
aortic valve endocarditis
aortic valve prosthesis (see *prosthesis*)

aortic valve replacement (AVR)
aortic window node
aorticopulmonary shunt; window
aortitis
  Döhle-Heller (or Doehle)
  giant cell
  luetic
  nummular
  rheumatic
  syphilitic
  Takayasu
aortitis syphilitica
aortoarteritis, nonspecific
aortobifemoral bypass; graft
aortocarotid bypass
aortocoronary bypass
aortocoronary snake graft
aortofemoral bypass graft (AFBG)
aortogram, aortography
  abdominal
  arch
  contrast
  digital subtraction supravalvular
  flush
  retrograde femoral
  retrograde transaxillary
  supravalvular
  thoracic arch
  translumbar
aortogram with distal runoff
aortoiliac aneurysm
aortoiliac occlusive disease
aortoiliofemoral bypass
aortoiliofemoral endarterectomy
aortopathy, idiopathic medial
aortoplasty, patch-graft
aortopulmonary shunt
aortopulmonary tunnel
aortopulmonary window operation
aortotomy, curvilinear
aortovelography, transcutaneous
  (TAV)
aortoventriculoplasty
AP (accessory pathway)
Ap (apical)

APB (atrial premature beat)
APC (atrial premature contraction)
APD (action potential duration)
aperture
apex
   apical
   cardiac
   displaced left ventricular
   uptilted cardiac
   ventricular
apex cardiogram, -graphy (ACG)
apex cordis (of heart)
apex of ventricle
apheresis
apical four-chamber view
apical hypoperfusion on thallium scan
apical impulse
apical surface of heart
apicoseptal aneurysmectomy
aplasia
   red cell
   right ventricular myocardial
APM (anterior papillary muscle)
Apo A1 LDL-cholesterol subfraction
Apo A2 LDL-cholesterol subfraction
Apo B LDL-cholesterol subfraction
apolipoprotein
apparatus, valvular
appearance and exclusion, normal
appendage
   atrial
   left atrial (LAA)
   right atrial
   truncated atrial
apposition
approach
   cephalic
   external jugular
   groin
   internal jugular
   percutaneous transfemoral

approach *(cont.)*
   subcostal
   subxiphoid
   transdiaphragmatic
   transxiphoid pacemaker lead
approximate, loosely
approximator
   Lemmon sternal
   Pilling Wolvek sternal
   Wolvek sternal
APSAC (anisoylated plasminogen streptokinase activator complex)
APT (atrial paroxysmal tachycardia)
Apt test
APTT (activated partial thromboplastin time)
AR (atrial rate; aortic regurgitation)
AR-2 diagnostic catheter
AR-2 guiding catheter
Arani double loop guiding catheter
arborization
arcade, septal
arcade of collaterals
arch
   aortic
   bifid aortic
   double aortic
   hypoplastic
   right aortic
   right-sided
   transverse
   transverse aortic
   Zimmerman
arch and carotid arteriography
arching of mitral valve leaflet
Arco pacemaker
Arcolithium pacemaker
arcus, corneal
area
   aortic
   aortic valve (AVA)
   arrhythmogenic
   artery
   Bamberger
   body surface (BSA)

area *(cont.)*
   cardiac frontal
   cross-sectional (CSA)
   effective balloon dilated (EBDA)
   Erb
   midsternal
   mitral valve (MVA)
   pulmonic
   stenosis
   tricuspid
   valve
area-length method for ejection
   fraction
argon laser
Argyle Sentinel Seal chest tube
Army-Navy retractor
ARP (absolute refractory period)
arrest
   cardiac
   cardioplegic
   cardiorespiratory
   circulatory
   cold cardioplegia
   deep hypothermic circulatory
   heart
   hypothermic fibrillating
   intermittent sinus
   sinus
   transient sinus
arrhythmia
   atrioventricular junctional
   AV nodal Wenckebach
   baseline
   continuous
   exercise-aggravated
   exercise-induced
   high-density ventricular
   inducible
   juvenile
   life-threatening
   malignant ventricular
   nodal
   nonrespiratory sinus
   pacing-induced termination of
   paroxysmal supraventricular

arrhythmia *(cont.)*
   perpetual
   phasic
   postperfusion
   reentrant
   reperfusion
   respiratory sinus
   sinus
   spontaneous
   stress-related
arrhythmia circuit
arrhythmia focus
Arrhythmia Net arrhythmia
   monitor
arrhythmogenic area of ventricle
arrhythmogenic right ventricular
   dysplasia
arrhythmogenic ventricular activity
   (AVA)
Arrow-Berman balloon angioplasty
   catheter
Arrow-Howes multi-lumen catheter
Arrow pulmonary artery catheter
arteria lusoria
arterial (ART)
arterial aneurysm
arterial blood gas (ABG) (see *blood gas)*
arterial cannula
arterial line (A line)
arterial oxygen saturation (SaO$_2$)
arterial pressure
arterial pulsation
arterial sheath
arteriogram, arteriography
   aorta and runoff
   arch
   biplane pelvic
   biplane quantitative coronary
   carotid
   cine
   coronary
   biplane pelvic
   Judkins technique for coronary
   left coronary cine

arteriogram *(cont.)*
  longitudinal
  percutaneous femoral
  pulmonary artery
  renal
  selective coronary
  Sones selective coronary
arteriola, arteriolae
arteriolar narrowing
arteriolar resistance
arteriole (arteriola)
arteriolith
arteriolitis
arteriolonecrosis
arteriolosclerosis
arteriomalacia
arteriometer
arteriomotor
arteriomyomatosis
arteriopathy
  hypertensive
  plexogenic pulmonary (PPA)
  thrombotic pulmonary (TPA)
arterioplasty
arteriorenal
arteriosclerosis
  cerebral
  coronary
  hyaline
  hypertensive
  infantile
  intimal
  medial
  Mönckeberg (Moenckeberg)
  peripheral
  senile
arteriosclerosis obliterans (ASO)
arteriosclerotic cardiovascular disease (ASCVD)
arteriosclerotic heart disease (ASHD)
arteriosclerotic peripheral vascular disease
arteriotomy, brachial
arteriovenous aneurysm
arteriovenous malformation (AVM)
arteriovenous oxygen difference (AVD O$_2$)
arteritis
  brachiocephalic
  coronary
  cranial
  giant cell
  granulomatous
  Horton
  infantile
  infectious
  localized visceral
  rheumatic
  syphilitic
  Takayasu
  temporal
  tuberculous
arteritis obliterans
arteritis umbilicalis
artery (see also *branch*)
  aberrant coronary
  anomalous origin of
  anterior descending branch of left coronary
  anterior inferior communicating (AICA)
  AV nodal
  beading of
  brachial
  brachiocephalic
  calcified
  circumflex (circ, CF, CX)
  circumflex coronary
  common carotid (CCA)
  conus
  diagonal branch of left anterior descending coronary
  descending septal
  diagonal coronary
  dilated
  distal circumflex marginal
  dominant coronary
  epicardial coronary
  external carotid

artery *(cont.)*
   external iliac
   high left main diagonal
   innominate
   intercostal
   intermediate coronary
   internal carotid (ICA)
   internal iliac
   internal mammary (IMA)
   Kugel
   LAD (left anterior descending)
   LAD coronary
   LCA (left coronary)
   LCF or LCX (left circumflex)
   left circumflex coronary
   left coronary (LCA)
   left internal mammary (LIMA)
   left main coronary (LMCA)
   left pulmonary (LPA)
   LIMA (left internal mammary)
   LMCA (left main coronary)
   main pulmonary (MPA)
   mainstem coronary
   marginal branch of left circumflex coronary
   marginal branch of right coronary
   marginal circumflex
   obtuse marginal
   PDA (posterior descending)
   popliteal
   posterior descending (PDA)
   posterior descending branch of right coronary
   posterior descending coronary
   posterior inferior communicating (PICA)
   profunda femoris
   proximal anterior descending
   proximal left anterior descending
   pulmonary (PA)
   ramus intermedius
   reperfused
   right coronary (RCA)
   right pulmonary (RPA)

artery *(cont.)*
   right ventricular branch of right coronary
   septal perforator
   sinus nodal
   stenotic coronary
   subclavian
   superficial femoral (SFA)
artifact
   baseline
   pacemaker
   pacing
artifactual
artificial blood
artificial heart (see *heart)*
artificial pacemaker
Arvidsson dimension-length method for ventricular volume
Arzco pacemaker
Arzco TAPSUL pill electrode
AS (aortic stenosis)
ASCD (aborted sudden cardiac death)
ascending aorta (AA)
Aschner phenomenon
Aschoff body; cell; node
Aschoff-Tawara node
ascorbate dilution curve
ASCVD (arterio- or atherosclerotic cardiovascular disease)
ASD (atrial septal defect)
ASH (asymmetric septal hypertrophy)
ASHD (arteriosclerotic heart disease)
Ashman beat
Ashman phenomenon
ASO (arteriosclerosis obliterans)
ASO titer test
aspartate aminotransferase (AST)
aspiration of air
aspirin, prophylactic use of
ASPVD (atherosclerotic pulmonary vascular disease)

assessment
   invasive
   noninvasive
assumed Fick method for cardiac output
AST (aspartate aminotransferase)
asthma, cardiac
Astra pacemaker
Astrand treadmill
ASTZ (antistreptozyme) test
ASVIP (atrial synchronous ventricular inhibited pacemaker)
asymmetric hypertrophy of septum
asymmetric septal hypertrophy (ASH)
asymmetry, facial
asynchronism
asynchrony
asyneresis
asynergy
   infarct-localized
   left ventricular
   regional
   segmental
asystole
   Beau
   cardiac
   complete atrial and ventricular
   ventricular
atherectomized vessel
atherectomy, retrograde
atherectomy cutter
atherectomy device, PET balloon Simpson
atherogenesis
atheroma, atheromatous
atheroembolism
atheroma
atheromatous debris; material
atheromatous plaque
atherosclerosis, intimal
atherosclerotic cardiovascular disease (ASCVD)
atherosclerotic narrowing
atherosclerotic plaque

ATL (anterior tricuspid leaflet)
Atlas LP PTCA balloon dilatation catheter
Atlas ULP balloon dilatation catheter
atmospheres of pressure
atresia
   aortic
   mitral
   pulmonary
   tricuspid
   ventricular
atretic
atria, atrial, atrium
atrial activation mapping, retrograde
atrial activation time
atrial cuff
atrial ectopy
atrial effective refractory period
atrial fibrillation (AF) with rapid ventricular response
atrial flutter (AFl)
atrial kick
atrial lead
atrial natriuretic factor (ANF)
atrial natriuretic polypeptide (ANP)
atrial overdrive pacing
atrial pacing wire, temporary
atrial paroxysmal tachycardia (APT)
atrial rate (AR)
atrial repolarization wave
atrial septal defect (ASD)
atrial single and double extrastimulation
atrial standstill
atrialized ventricle
Atricor pacemaker
atriofascicular tract
atriography, negative contrast left
atrio-His pathway; tract
atrio-Hisian bypass tract; fiber
atriotomy
atrioventricular (AV) canal
atrioventricular dissociation
atrioventricular junction

atrioventricular nodal rhythm
atrioventricular nodal tachycardia
atrioventricular ring
atrioventricular septal defect
atrioventricular time
atrium, atria, atrial
atrium
  common
  high right
  left (LA)
  low septal right
  pulmonary
  right (RA)
Atrium Blood Recovery System
atrium cordis
atrium dextrum
atrium pulmonale
atrium sinistrum
atropine via endotracheal tube
attack
  heart
  Stokes-Adams
attenuate
atypical chest pain
augmented EKG leads
auricle
auricular rate
Aurora dual-chamber pacemaker
Aurora pulse generator
auscultation and percussion
auscultatory gap
Austin Flint murmur
Austin Flint phenomenon
Austin Flint rumble (murmur)
Autima II pacemaker
autoclaved, steam
autologous blood transfusion
autologous vein graft
automatic implantable (or internal) cardioverter defibrillator (AICD)
automatic implantable defibrillator (AID)
automaticity
  enhanced
  pacemaker

automaticity *(cont.)*
  sinus node
  triggered
Autoplex Factor VIII inhibitor bypass product
Auto-Suture surgical stapler
autotransfusion system
AV (aortic valve) repair
AV (arterial/venous) oxygen difference
AV (arteriovenous or atrioventricular) block (see *block)*
AV bundle in the heart
AV conduction defect
AV disable mechanism of pacemaker
AVDH (AV delay hysteresis)
AVDI (AV delay interval)
AV dissociation, isorhythmic
AV groove
AV junctional escape beat; complex
AV junctional rhythm
AV nodal pathway
AV nodal reentry tachycardia
AV nodal rhythm
AV nodal Wenckebach arrhythmia
AV node conduction abnormality
AV reciprocating tachycardia
AV sequential pacing
AV valve
AVA (aortic valve area; arrhythmogenic ventricular activity)
AVCO aortic balloon
AVD (aortic valvular disease)
AVD (atrioventricular dissociation)
AVD O_2 (arteriovenous oxygen difference)
aV_F or aVF (augmented lead, left foot) EKG lead
AVF (arteriovenous fistula)
AVG (aortic valve gradient)
Avitene topical hemostatic material
Avius sequential pacemaker
aV_L or aVL (augmented lead, left arm) EKG lead

AVM (arteriovenous or atrioventricular malformation)
AVNR (atrioventricular nodal
  rhythm)
AVNRT (atrioventricular nodal reentrant tachycardia)
AVNT (atrioventricular nodal
  tachycardia)
AV O_2 difference
  pulmonary
  systemic
AVP (ambulant venous pressure)
AVR (aortic valve replacement)
aV_R or avR (augmented lead,
  right arm) EKG lead
AVRT (atrioventricular reciprocating tachycardia)
AVSD (acquired ventricular septal
  defect)
axillobifemoral bypass
Axiom DG balloon angioplasty
  catheter
axis
  arterial
  clockwise rotation of electrical
  electrical
  heart
  J point electrical
  junctional
  left
  mean electrical
  mean QRS
  normal
  P wave
  right
  superior QRS
  twisting on the electrical
  variable
axis deviation
  horizontal
  left
  vertical
axis of EKG lead
Ayerza syndrome

B

B bump on echocardiogram
B-mode (B-scan)
Bachmann bundle
Bachmann, pathway of
back-bleeding
backflow from arterial line
Baffe anastomosis
baffle
  intra-atrial
  pericardial
  Senning type of intra-atrial
baffle leak
bag
  Ambu
  Douglas
  manual resuscitation
bagged (ventilated)
Bahnson aortic clamp
Bailey aortic clamp
Bailey aortic valve cutting forceps
Bailey rib contractor; spreader
Bailey-Gibbon rib contractor
Bailey-Glover-O'Neill commissur-
  otomy knife
bailout catheter; valvuloplasty
Baim catheter
Baim-Turi monitoring/pacing
  catheter
BAL (bronchoalveolar lavage)
Balke treadmill exercise protocol
Balke-Ware treadmill exercise
  protocol

ball poppet of prosthetic valve
ball-wedge
ballistocardiography
balloon
   ACS SULP II
   AVCO aortic
   catheter
   counterpulsation
   Hartzler angioplasty
   intra-aortic (IAB)
   kissing
   Kontron intra-aortic
   LPS
   Mansfield
   Percor DL-II (dual-lumen) intra-aortic
   Percor-Stat intra-aortic
   PET
balloon inflation
balloon-tipped catheter
Bamberger sign
band
   CPK-MB
   CPK-MM
   parietal
bandage, Esmarch
banding, pulmonary artery
Bannister disease
Bard arterial cannula
Bard Cardiopulmonary Support System
Bard guiding catheter
Bard-Parker knife
Bardic cannula
Bardic cutdown catheter
barium-impregnated poppet
Barlow syndrome
baroreceptor, carotid
baroreflex
   carotid
   sinoatrial
barrel-chested
barrier, blood-brain
base of heart
baseline artifact

baseline of EKG
baseline ST segment abnormality
baseline standing blood pressure
baseline standing pulse rate
basic cardiac life support (BCLS)
basic cycle length (BCL)
basic drive cycle length (BDCL)
basic rate
Basix pacemaker
basket, pericardial
battery, external pacemaker
battery voltage
bat's wing shadow on x-ray
Bayes theorem
BBB (bundle branch block)
BBBB (bilateral bundle branch block)
BBR (bundle branch reentry)
BCL (basic cycle length)
BCLS (basic cardiac life support)
BDCL (basic drive cycle length)
beading of artery
Beall circumflex artery scissors
Beall disk valve prosthesis
Beall mitral valve prosthesis
Beall prosthetic valve
Beall-Surgitool ball-cage prosthetic valve
Beall-Surgitool disk prosthetic valve
beat (see also *heartbeat*)
   aberrantly conducted
   apex
   Ashman
   asynchronous
   atrial escape
   atrial fusion
   atrial premature (APB)
   AV junctional escape
   capture
   dropped
   echo
   ectopic ventricular
   entrained
   escape
   forced

beat *(cont.)*
  fusion
  interpolated
  junctional escape
  malignant
  missed
  postectopic
  premature atrial (PAB)
  premature ventricular (PVB)
  pseudofusion
  reciprocal
  skipped
  sustained ventricular apex
  ventricular ectopic (VEB)
  ventricular escape
  ventricular premature (VPB)
beat, entrained
beat-to-beat variability
beating at a fixed rate
beats per minute (BPM or bpm)
Beau asystole; disease
Beaver blade; knife
Beck miniature aortic clamp
Beck vascular clamp
Beck-Potts clamp
Beckman O_2 analyzer
Beckman retractor
Becton Dickinson Teflon-sheathed needle
bed
  capillary
  pulmonary
bedside commode
beep-o-gram
bell of stethoscope
Bengolea artery forceps
Bentall inclusion technique
Bentall operation
Bentley oxygenator
Bentley transducer
Bentson guide wire
Berenstein catheter
Berman angiographic catheter
Berman aortic clamp
Bernheim syndrome
Bernoulli equation; theorem
Bernstein study
berry aneurysm
Berry sternal needle holder
beta-adrenergic blocking agent
$beta_1$-adrenergic receptor
$beta_2$-adrenergic receptor
beta-adrenoreceptor blocking agent
beta antagonist
beta blockade; blocker
beta lipoprotein fraction
beta-thromboglobulin
Bethune rib shears
Bethune rongeur
bevel, beveled, beveling
Bezold-Jarisch reflex
biatrial myxoma
bibasilar crackles
BICAP unit
bicaval cannulation
Biceps bipolar coagulator
bicuspid aortic valve
bicycle
  Aerobicycle
  Aerodyne
  Collins
  Siemens-Albis
  Tredex powered
bicycle ergometer
bicycle exercise test
bidirectional
bifascicular block
bifid
bifurcate, bifurcation
bifurcation
  carotid
  iliac
bigeminal rhythm
bigeminy
bigeminy bisferious pulse (pulsus bisferiens)
BIMA (bilateral internal mammary artery) reconstruction)
bioimpedance, thoracic electrical (TEB)

Biomer (segmented polyurethane)
Bionit vascular prosthesis
biophysical profile (BPP)
bioprosthesis (see *prosthesis)*
Biotronik pacemaker
biphasic
biphasic complex on EKG
biphasic P wave
biplane pelvic arteriography
biplane pelvic oblique study
bipolar generator
bipolar lead
bipolar pacemaker
bipolar temporary pacemaker
   catheter
Bisping electrode
biventricular hypertrophy
Bivona tracheostomy tube
Bjork-Shiley aortic valve prosthesis
Blackfan-Diamond syndrome
blade
   Bard-Parker
   Beaver
   electrosurgical
   knife
Blalock pulmonary clamp
Blalock shunt
Blalock-Hanlon operation
Blalock-Niedner clamp
Blalock-Taussig operation
Blalock-Taussig shunt
blanket, hypothermia
bleeding time (see *time)*
block
   2:1; 3:2
   acquired symptomatic AV
   arborization
   arteriovenous (AV)
   atrioventricular (AV)
   AV (arteriovenous; atrio-
      ventricular)
   AV Wenckebach heart
   BBB (bundle branch)
   BBBB (bilateral bundle branch)
   bifascicular

block *(cont.)*
   bifascicular bundle branch
   bilateral bundle branch (BBBB)
   bundle branch (BBB)
   complete AV (CAVB)
   complete heart (CHB)
   congenital heart
   congenital symptomatic AV
   entrance
   exit
   familial heart
   fascicular
   first-degree atrioventricular (AV)
   first-degree heart
   fixed third-degree AV
   heart
   high-degree AV
   incomplete atrioventricular
      (IAVB)
   incomplete left bundle branch
      (ILBBB)
   incomplete right bundle branch
      (IRBBB)
   inflammatory heart
   infra-His
   intermittent third-degree AV
   intra-atrial
   intra-His; intra-Hisian
   intranodal
   intraventricular conduction
   ipsilateral bundle branch
   left anterior fascicular (LAFB)
   left bundle branch (LBBB)
   left posterior fascicular (LPFB)
   Mobitz I or II second-degree AV
   Mobitz type I on Wenckebach
      heart
   paroxysmal AV
   peri-infarction (PIB)
   pseudo-AV
   right bundle branch (RBBB)
   second-degree AV
   second-degree heart
   sinoatrial (SAB)
   sinoatrial exit

block *(cont.)*
  sinus
  sinus exit
  sinus node exit
  supra-Hisian
  third-degree AV
  transient AV
  trifascicular
  VA (ventriculoatrial)
  ventricular
  Wenckebach AV
Block right coronary guiding catheter
blockade, alpha-adrenergic
blocked APC (atrial premature contraction)
blocker
  beta
  $alpha_1$-adrenergic
  calcium channel
  slow channel
blood
  arterial
  artificial
  autologous
  cord
  defibrinated
  deoxygenated
  frank
  heparinized
  laky
  occult
  oxygenated
  peripheral
  shunted
  sludged
  unoxygenated
  venous
  whole
blood-brain barrier
blood clot
blood coagulation factors (see *factors*)
blood flow on Doppler echocardiogram

blood gas (arterial), *consisting of:*
  base excess
  bicarbonate
  HCO_3
  O_2 saturation (%)
  $PaCO_2$
  PaO_2
  pCO_2
  pH
  pO_2
  venous
blood gases on oxygen
blood gases on room air
bloodless fluid
blood pool
blood pressure (BP)
  baseline
  baseline standing
  high
  low
  orthostatic
  standing
  supine
  systolic/diastolic
blood pressure response
blood sample
bloodstream
blood urea nitrogen (BUN)
Bloodwell forceps
Bloom DTU 201 external stimulator
Bloom programmable stimulator
blue baby
blue finger syndrome
Blue Max triple-lumen catheter
blue toe syndrome ("trash foot")
BML (billowing mitral leaflet)
body
  Aschoff
  gelatin compression
  Heinz
Boettcher artery forceps
bolster, Teflon felt
bolus intravenous injection
bolus of medication
bone wax

booming diastolic rumble
boot
  sheepskin
  Unna
border
  cardiac
  lower sternal (LSB)
  upper sternal
Borg scale of treadmill exertion
Bornholm disease
Bosch ERG 500 ergometer
Bouillaud disease; sign; syndrome
bouts of tachycardia
Bouveret disease
bovine allograft; heterograft
bovine pericardial bioprosthesis
bowing of mitral valve leaflet
Boyd perforating vein
Bozzolo sign
BP (blood pressure)
BPM or bpm (beats per minute)
BPP (biophysical profile)
BPV (balloon pulmonary valvuloplasty)
brachial artery
brachial pulse
brachiocephalic trunk
Bradbury-Eggleston syndrome
bradyarrhythmia, digitalis-induced
bradycardia
  Branham
  central
  essential
  idioventricular
  intermittent junctional
  junctional
  nodal
  postinfective
  pulseless
  sinoatrial
  sinus (SB)
  vagal
bradycardia-tachycardia syndrome
bradydysrhythmia
bradykinin

bradysphygmia
bradytachycardia syndrome
bradytachydysrhythmia syndrome
branch (see also *artery*)
  acute marginal
  AV groove
  bifurcating
  diagonal
  first diagonal
  first major diagonal
  first septal perforator
  inferior wall
  left bundle
  marginal
  obtuse marginal (OMB)
  posterior descending
  ramus
  right bundle
  septal
  septal perforating
  side
  ventricular
branching, mirror-image brachiocephalic
Branham sign
Brasdor method
Braunwald sign
Braunwald-Cutter ball prosthetic valve
brawny edema
breathlessness
Brechenmacher fiber; tract
Brescio-Cimino AV (arteriovenous) fistula
bridging, muscular
Broadbent inverted sign
Brock cardiac dilator
Brock clamp
Brock commissurotomy knife
Brockenbrough catheter, modified bipolar
Brockenbrough mapping catheter
Brockenbrough needle
Brockenbrough sign
Brockenbrough transseptal catheter

Brockenbrough transseptal method
   for commissurotomy
Broncho-Cath endotracheal tube
Broviac atrial catheter
Brown Adson forceps
Brown-Dodge method for
   angiography
Bruce protocol
   modified
   standard
   treadmill exercise
bruit, bruits
   aneurysmal
   audible
   carotid
   epigastric
   false
   flank
   palpable
   renal artery
   Roger
   sea gull (or sea-gull)
   subclavian
   supraclavicular
   systolic
   Traube
bruit de canon
bruit de choc
bruit de craquement
bruit de cuir neuf
bruit de diable
bruit de fêlé
bruit de frolement
bruit de frottement
bruit de galop
bruit de lime
bruit de moulin
bruit de parchemin
bruit de piaulement
bruit de rape
bruit de rappel
bruit de Roger
bruit de scie
bruit de soufflet
bruit de tabourka
bruit de tambour
bruit de triolet
Brunschwig artery forceps
BSA (body surface area)
BSA ejection fraction
Buchbinder Omniflex catheter
Buchbinder Thruflex catheter
Buchbinder Thruflex Over-the-Wire
buckling of mitral valve, midsystolic
Buerger disease
Buerger-Gruetz disease
buffer
bulb
   aortic
   carotid
bulldog clamp
BUN (blood urea nitrogen)
bundle
   AV (atrioventricular)
   Bachmann
   His
   James
   Keith sinoatrial
   Kent
   Kent-His
   Mahaim
   main
   sinoatrial
   Thorel
bundle branch block (BBB)
bundle branch reentry (BBR)
bundle of His
bundle of Stanley Kent
Burford retractor
Burford rib spreader
Burford-Finochietto rib spreader
burr, atherectomy
burst of arrhythmia
burst of pacing
burst of ventricular ectopy
burst of ventricular tachycardia
butterfly, silicone
butterfly shadow on x-ray
buttock claudication
button, skin

button of aorta
button technique
BVAD (biventricular assist device), Thoratec
BV-2 needle
bypass (see also *graft*)
  aorta to first obtuse marginal branch
  aorta to LAD
  aorta to marginal branch
  aorta to posterior descending
  aortic-femoral
  aortobifemoral
  aortobi-iliac
  aortocarotid
  aortocoronary-saphenous vein
  aortofemoral
  aortoiliofemoral
  aorto-subclavian-carotid-axilloaxillary
  atrial-femoral artery
  axillary
  axilloaxillary
  axillobifemoral
  axillofemoral
  brachial
  cardiopulmonary (CPB)
  carotid-axillary
  carotid-carotid
  carotid-subclavian
  coronary artery (CAB)
  cross femoral-femoral crossover
  DTAF-F (descending thoracic aortofemoral-femoral)
  fem-fem (femoral-femoral)

bypass *(cont.)*
  femoral crossover
  femoral-popliteal
  femoral-tibial-peroneal
  femoral to tibial
  femoral vein-femoral artery
  femoroaxillary
  femorodistal
  femorofemoral crossover
  femoropopliteal saphenous vein
  femorotibial
  fem-pop (femoral-popliteal)
  heart-lung
  iliopopliteal
  infracubital
  in situ
  ipsilateral nonreversed greater saphenous vein
  left atrium to distal arterial aortic
  Litwak left atrial-aortic
  partial cardiopulmonary
  percutaneous femoral-femoral cardiopulmonary
  pulsatile cardiopulmonary
  renal artery–reverse saphenous vein
  reversed
  subclavian-carotid
  subclavian-subclavian
  superior mesenteric artery
  temporary aortic shunt
  total cardiopulmonary
bypass circuit
Byrel SX pacemaker
Byrel-SX/Versatrax pacemaker

C

C point of cardiac apex pulse
c wave of jugular venous pulse
c wave pressure on right atrial catheterization
C-11 palmitate uptake on PET scan
C-A (cardiac-apnea) monitor for newborns
C-A amplitude of mitral valve
CADS (computer-assisted diagnostics)
C-C (convexo-concave) heart valve
C'H$_{50}$ (total hemolytic complement)
CAB (coronary artery bypass)
"cabbage" (CABG)
CABG (coronary artery bypass graft)
cable
  alligator pacing
  fibrillator
  percutaneous
Cabot-Locke murmur
CABS (coronary artery bypass surgery)
cachexia, cardiac
CAD (coronary artery disease)
calcific spur
calcification
  annular
  coronary
  dystrophic
  linear
  mitral annular
  Mönckeberg (Moenckeberg)
  subannular
  valve
  valvular
calcification of pericardium
calcification of valve
calcified valvular leaflets
calcium antagonist
calcium channel blocker
calcium deposit

caliber of vessel
  borderline
  suitable
Calman carotid artery clamp
Calman ring clamp
camera
  Anger-type scintillation
  multicrystal gamma
CAMV (congenital anomaly of mitral valve)
canal
  arterial
  atrioventricular (AV)
  common atrioventricular
  complex atrioventricular
  Hunter
  pulmoaortic
canal of Cuvier
Cannon "a" wave of jugular venous pulse
cannula, cannulae, cannulas
  aortic arch
  arterial
  atrial
  Bard arterial
  Bardic
  Cope needle introducer
  coronary artery
  coronary perfusion
  femoral artery
  Gregg-type
  high-flow
  infusion
  inlet
  intra-arterial
  Litwak
  LV (left ventricular) apex
  metallic tip
  nasal (for oxygen)
  outlet
  perfusion
  Polystan perfusion

cannula *(cont.)*
   Portnoy ventricular
   Sarns aortic arch
   Sarns two-stage
   Sarns venous drainage
   Storz needle
   two-stage Sarns
   vena cava
   Venflon
   venous
   ventricular
   washout
   Webster infusion
cannulate, percutaneously
cannulated
cannulation, cannulization
   bicaval
   ostial
capacity
   cardiac functional
   O_2 carrying
Capetown aortic prosthetic valve
capillary bed
capillary bud
capillary filling, compensatory
capillary filtration coefficient (CFC)
capillary refill
Capiox-E bypass system oxygenator
capture
   failure to
   lack of pacemaker
   loss of
   1:1 retrograde
   pacemaker
   resistance
   retrograde atrial
CAR (carotid arterial) pulse
carbon-11 palmitic acid radioactive tracer
carcinoid heart disease
Cardarelli sign
cardiac apex
cardiac arrest
cardiac asthma
cardiac blood pool imaging

cardiac catheterization
cardiac cirrhosis
cardiac cycle
cardiac dilation
cardiac efficiency
cardiac enlargement
cardiac enzymes (see *isoenzymes*)
cardiac fossa
cardiac function
cardiac functional capacity
cardiac index (CI)
cardiac glycoside
cardiac isoenzymes (see *isoenzymes*)
cardiac leads (see *lead*)
cardiac massage
cardiac output (CO) (see *output*)
cardiac rehabilitation program
cardiac reserve
cardiac rhythm disturbance
cardiac risk factor (see *risk factors*)
cardiac shunt
cardiac silhouette (on x-ray)
cardiac source
Cardiac Stimulator BCO_2
cardiac surgery intensive care unit (CSICU)
cardiac tamponade
cardiac thrust
cardiac transplant recipient (CTR)
cardiac valvar operation
cardiac waist
cardiac-apnea (CA) monitor for newborns
cardialgia
cardiectasis
cardioangiography
cardioangioscope, Sumida
cardiocentesis
Cardio Data MK-3 Holter scanner
CardioDiary heart monitor
cardiodynia
cardiogenic shock
cardiogram, cardiography
   apex (ACG)
   esophageal

cardiogram *(cont.)*
   precordial
   ultrasonic (UCG)
   vector
Cardio-Green dye
cardiointegram (CIG)
cardiokymographic (CKG) test
cardiologist
cardiomegaly, globular
cardiomyoliposis
cardiomyopathic lentiginosis
cardiomyopathy
   alcoholic
   apical hypertrophic (AHC)
   beer-drinker's
   concentric hypertrophic
   congestive
   constrictive
   diabetic
   dilated (DCM)
   end-stage
   familial hypertrophic (FHC)
   hypertrophic (HCM)
   hypertrophic obstructive (HOC or HOCM)
   idiopathic dilated (IDC)
   infiltrative
   ischemic
   nonischemic congestive
   nonobstructive
   obstructive hypertrophic
   peripartum
   postpartum
   primary
   restricted (RCM)
   restrictive
   secondary
   tachycardia-induced
   viral
cardiomyopathy with restrictive component
cardio-omentopexy
Cardio-Pace Medical Durapulse pacemaker
cardiopathy, infarctoid
cardiopericardiopexy
cardiopericarditis
cardiophrenic angle
cardioplegia (see also *solution*)
   cold
   cold blood
   cold potassium
   cold sanguineous
   crystalloid potassium
   hyperkalemic
   nutrient
   potassium chloride
cardioplegic needle
cardioplegic solution (cardioplegia)
cardioprotective
cardioptosis, Wenckebach
cardiopulmonary bypass (CPB)
cardiopulmonary resuscitation (CPR)
cardioselective agent
cardioselective beta blocker
cardioscope U system
cardiospasm
cardiotachometer
cardiothoracic ratio (CTR)
cardiothoracic surgeon
cardiothyrotoxicosis
cardiotomy
cardiotoxicity
   Adriamycin
   doxorubicin
cardiovalvulitis
cardiovascular hemodynamics
cardiovascular steady state
cardiovascular tone
cardioversion
   DC (direct-current)
   endocavitary
   synchronized DC
cardiovert, attempt to
cardioverted
cardioverter-defibrillator, automatic implantable (AICD)
cardioverter-defibrillator, implantable

carditis
  rheumatic
  streptococcal
  verrucous
Carey Coombs murmur
Carmalt forceps
carotid baroreceptor
carotid bulb
carotid bruit
carotid ejection time
carotid endarterectomy
carotid massage
carotid occlusive disease
carotid pulse
carotid shudder
carotid sinus hypersensitivity (CSH)
carotid sinus massage
carotid sinus syncope
carotid sinus syndrome
carotid upstroke, brisk
carotid-subclavian bypass
carotids, equal
Carpentier annuloplasty ring prosthesis
Carpentier ring
Carpentier tricuspid valvuloplasty
Carpentier-Edwards aortic valve
Carpentier-Edwards bioprosthetic valve
Carpentier-Edwards mitral annuloplasty valve
Carpentier-Edwards pericardial valve
Carpentier-Edwards Porcine SupraAnnular (SAV) valve
Carrel patch
Carter equation
Carvallo sign
CAS (coronary artery spasm)
CASE computerized exercise EKG system
CASS criteria
Castaneda anastomosis clamp
Castaneda vascular clamp
Castellino sign
Castillo catheter

CAT (computerized axial tomography)
catadicrotic pulse
cath (catheterization)
cathed (catheterized)
catheter
  ACS (Advanced Catheter or Cardiovascular Systems)
  ACS JL4 (Judkins left 4 French)
  ACS Mini
  ACS RX coronary dilatation
  Amplatz cardiac
  Amplatz femoral
  Amplatz right coronary
  angiographic balloon occlusion
  Angio-Kit
  angiopigtail
  angioplasty balloon
  Angled Balloon
  angulated
  Anthron heparinized aortogram
  AR-2 diagnostic; guiding
  Arani double loop guiding
  Arrow pulmonary artery
  Arrow-Berman balloon
  Arrow-Howes multi-lumen
  arterial embolectomy
  atherectomy, peripheral
  Atlas LP PTCA balloon dilatation
  Atlas ULP balloon dilatation
  Axiom DG balloon angioplasty
  bailout
  Baim
  Baim-Turi monitor/pacing
  balloon dilatation
  balloon dilating
  balloon embolectomy
  balloon flotation
  balloon septostomy
  balloon-tipped angiographic
  balloon-tipped, flow-directed
  Bard guiding
  Bardic cutdown

catheter *(cont.)*
Berenstein
Berman angiograpic
bipolar pacing electrode
bipolar temporary pacemaker
Block right coronary guiding
Blue Max triple-lumen
Brockenbrough mapping
Brockenbrough modified bipolar
Brockenbrough transseptal
Broviac atrial
Buchbinder Omniflex
Buchbinder Thruflex
cardiac
Castillo
central venous
Cloverleaf
coaxial
Cobra
cobra-shaped
coil-tipped
conductance
Cook arterial
Cook pigtail
Cordis Brite Tip guiding
Cordis high-flow pigtail
coronary dilatation
coronary guiding
coronary sinus thermodilution
Cournand
Critikon
cryoablation
cutdown
CVP (central venous pressure)
Dacron
diagnostic
dilatation balloon
dilating
DLP cardioplegic
Doppler coronary
Dorros brachial internal mammary guiding
Dotter caged balloon
Dotter coaxial
double-lumen

catheter *(cont.)*
Ducor balloon
DVI Simpson atherocath
Edwards diagnostic
El Gamal coronary bypass
Elecath thermodilution
embolectomy
end-hole
Enhanced Torque 8F guiding
Eppendorf
extrusion balloon
FAST (flow-assisted, short-term) balloon
femoral guiding
Finesse large-lumen guiding
flotation
flow-directed
flow-oximetry
fluid-filled
Fogarty arterial embolectomy
Fogarty balloon
Fogarty occlusion
Fogarty venous thrombectomy
Fogarty-Chin extrusion balloon
French 5 (5 French) angiographic
French MBIH
Ganz-Edwards coronary infusion
Gensini
Gentle-Flo suction
Goodale-Lubin
Gorlin
Gould PentaCath 5-lumen thermodilution
graft-seeking
Grollman
Groshong double-lumen
Gruentzig arterial balloon
Gruentzig Dilaca
guiding
Hanafee
Hartzler LPS dilatation
Hartzler Micro II
Hartzler Micro XT dilatation
headhunter visceral angiography
hexapolar

catheter *(cont.)*
- Hickman indwelling right atrial
- Hidalgo
- high-flow
- high-fidelity
- hot-tip
- HydraCross TLC PTCA
- IAB (intra-aortic balloon)
- indwelling
- Inoue balloon
- intra-aortic balloon
- intracath
- intracoronary guiding
- intracoronary perfusion
- intravenous pacing
- JL4, JR4 (Judkins left [or right] 4 cm)
- JL5, JR5 (Judkins left [or right] 5 cm)
- Judkins left (or right) coronary
- Judkins USCI
- Kensey atherectomy
- King multipurpose coronary graft
- large-bore
- large-lumen
- laser
- left ventricular sump
- Lehman ventriculography
- Longdwel Teflon
- Lo-Profile balloon
- Lo-Profile II balloon
- Lo-Profile steerable dilatation
- LPS
- Lumaguide
- Mallinckrodt angiographic
- Mansfield Scientific dilatation balloon
- McGoon coronary perfusion
- McIntosh double-lumen
- Meditech balloon
- Medtronic balloon
- Micro-Guide
- micromanometer-tip
- midstream aortogram
- Millar micromanometer

catheter *(cont.)*
- Millar pigtail angiographic
- Mini-Profile dilatation
- Mitsubishi angioscopic
- Monorail angioplasty
- MPF
- Mullins transseptal
- multi-electrode impedance
- Multi-Med triple-lumen infusion
- multi-lumen
- multipolar impedance
- multipurpose
- Myler
- NIH (National Institutes of Health)
- NIH left ventriculography
- Nycore angiography
- Omniflex balloon
- Optiscope
- oximetric
- oximetry
- Paceport
- pacing
- Pathfinder
- PE Plus II balloon dilatation
- Percor-DL
- Percor-Stat-DL
- percutaneous
- perfusion
- pervenous
- PIBC (percutaneous intra-aortic balloon counterpulsation)
- pigtail
- polyethylene
- Polystan venous return
- Positrol II
- preformed
- preshaped
- probing
- Profile Plus dilatation
- Proflex 5 dilatation
- PTCA
- pulmonary artery
- pulmonary flotation
- pulmonary triple-lumen

catheter *(cont.)*
quadripolar
Quanticor
Quinton
Raaf Cath vascular
radial artery
Rashkind balloon
Rashkind septostomy balloon
recessed balloon septostomy
RediFurl TaperSeal IAB
Rentrop infusion
retroperfusion
RF (radiofrequency-generated thermal) balloon
right coronary
Rodriguez
Royal Flush angiographic flush
Rumel
Schneider
Schneider-Shiley
Schoonmaker femoral
Schoonmaker multipurpose
Schwarten balloon dilatation
Sci-Med SSC "Skinny"
sensing
shaver
Sheldon
Shiley guiding
Shiley-Ionescu
SHJR4s (side-hole Judkins right, curve 4, short)
side-hole
sidewinder
Silastic
Silicore
Simmons-type (sidewinder)
Simplus PE/t dilatation
Simpson peripheral AtheroCath
Simpson Ultra Lo-Profile II balloon
Simpson-Robert
single-stage
Softip arteriography
Softip diagnostic
Softouch guiding

catheter *(cont.)*
Sones Cardio-Marker
Sones Hi-Flow
Sones Pistrol
Stack perfusion coronary dilatation
steerable
Stertzer brachial guiding
stimulating
straight flush percutaneous
SULP II
sump
Swan-Ganz balloon-flotation pulmonary artery
Swan-Ganz Guidewire TD
Swan-Ganz thermodilution
TAC atherectomy
Teflon
temporary pacing
Tennis Racquet angiographic
thermistor
thermodilution balloon
thermodilution pacing
thermodilution Swan-Ganz
thrombectomy
Thruflex PTCA balloon
toposcopic
Torcon NB selective angiographic
transducer-tipped
transluminal extraction (TEC)
transseptal
transvenous pacemaker
triple-lumen
triple thermistor coronary sinus
tripolar
Tygon
ULP (ultra low profile)
USCI Bard
USCI guiding
USCI Mini-Profile balloon dilatation
valvuloplasty balloon
Van Tassel pigtail
Variflex
venous thrombectomy

catheter *(cont.)*
  venting
  ventriculography
  Vitalcor venous
  Webster coronary sinus
  Williams L-R guiding
  Wilton-Webster coronary sinus
  Zucker
catheter advanced under fluoroscopic guidance
catheter bailout
catheter damping
catheter electrode
catheter exchanged over a guide wire
catheter sheath
catheter-skin interface
catheter tip
catheterization
  antegrade transseptal left heart
  cardiac
  central venous (CVC)
  left heart
  Mullins modification of transseptal
  PTCA
  retrograde
  retrograde left heart
  right heart
  selective cardiac
  simultaneous right and left heart
  transseptal heart
  transseptal left heart
catheterizing
cathode, epicardial patch
caudal view
cautery
caval snare
CAVB (complete atrioventricular block)
Caves-Schulz bioptome
cavity, pericardial
cavogram
CBC (complete blood cell count): hematocrit

CBC *(cont.)*
  hemoglobin
  MCH (mean corpuscular hemoglobin)
  MCHC (mean corpuscular hemoglobin concentration)
  MCV (mean corpuscular volume)
  RBC (red blood cell) count
  WBC (white blood cell) count
CBC with diff (differential)
CBC with WBC and differential
CBV (catheter balloon valvuloplasty)
C-C (convexo-concave) heart valve
C, C, or E (clubbing, cyanosis, or edema)
CCA (common carotid artery)
CCU (coronary care unit; critical care unit) protocol
CD (conduction defect)
C-E amplitude of mitral valve
CECG (continuous electrocardiographic monitoring)
Cedars-Sinai classification of pump failure
Cegka sign
cell
  adventitial
  Ashoff
  blood
  chicken-wire myocardial
  foamy myocardial
  Marchand
  P
  pacemaker
  perithelial
Cell Saver Haemonetics Autotransfusion System
celltrifuge
Cenflex central monitoring system
central aortic pressure
central intra-aortic pressure curve
central venous line
central venous pressure (CVP)
cephalad

cephalic vein
cephalization of pulmonary flow pattern
cerebrovascular accident (CVA) (stroke)
CFC (capillary filtration coefficient)
CFR (coronary flow reserve)
CGR biplane angiographic system
Chagas disease
chamber
  cardiac
  false aneurysmal
chamber compression
chamber of heart
chamber size
Chandler V-pacing probe
change, changes
  diagnostic ST segment
  EKG
  ischemic
  nonspecific
  T wave
  serial
  ST and T wave
channel
  blood
  central
  fast sodium
  slow calcium
  sodium
  thoroughfare
character of pulse
Charcot sign
Charcot-Bouchard aneurysm
Chardack-Greatbatch Implantable Cardiac Pulse Generator
Chardack-Greatbatch pacemaker
CHARGE syndrome
CHB (complete heart block)
CHD (congenital heart disease)
Check-Flo introducer
check-valve sheath
Chemo-Port
chest pain (see *angina*)
chest tube (see *tube*)

chest wall tenderness
chest x-ray (CXR), baseline
CHF (congestive heart failure; congenital heart failure)
Chiari syndrome
Chiari-Budd syndrome
chicken-wire myocardial cell
chloride, chlorides
cholesterol
  serum
  total plasma
cholesterol cleft
chordae
  elongation of
  shortening of
chordae tendineae, ruptured
chordal length
Chorus pacemaker
Christmas blood coagulation factor
Christmas disease (hemophilia B)
chronic atrial fibrillation with slow ventricular response
chronic hypertensive disease
chronic hyperventilation syndrome
chronic lead placement
Chronocor IV external pacemaker
chronotropic effect
chronotropic incompetence
chronotropic response; therapy
CHS (carotid sinus hypersensitivity)
Church scissors
chylomicron
chylomicronemia
CI (cardiac index)
Cibatome
CIG (cardiointegram)
cigarette smoking, pack-years of
cine CT (computed tomography) scanner
cineangiocardiography
cineangiogram, cineangiography
  biplane
  coronary
  left ventricular (LV)
  radionuclide

cineangiogram *(cont.)*
  selective coronary
    Sones technique for
cinefluorography
cinefluoroscopy
cineventriculogram, -graphy,
  biplane
circ, CF, CX (circumflex artery)
circadian event recorder
circle of Vieussens
circuit
  arrhythmia
  bypass
  shunting
circular plane
circulation
  allantoic
  assisted
  balanced coronary
  codominant coronary
  collateral
  compensatory
  derivative
  extracorporeal
  fetal
  greater
  intervillous
  left circumflex-dominant
  left-dominant coronary
  lesser
  peripheral
  placental
  portal
  pulmonary
  right-dominant coronary
  systemic
circulatory arrest
circulatory embarrassment
circulatory impairment
circulatory support
circumferential
circumflex coronary artery
circus movement
circus-movement tachycardia (CMT)
cirrhosis, cardiac

cirsodesis
CK/AST ratio
CKG (cardiokymographic) test
CK (creatine kinase) isoenzymes
  CK-BB fraction (CK_1)
  CK-MB fraction (CK_2)
  CK-MM fraction (CK_3)
clamp (also *clip*)
  Alfred M. Large vena cava
  Allis
  anastomosis
  angled peripheral vascular
  aortic aneurysm
  aortic occlusion
  appendage
  Bahnson aortic
  Bailey aortic
  Beck aortic
  Beck miniature aortic
  Beck vascular
  Beck-Potts
  Berman aortic
  Blalock pulmonary
  Blalock-Niedner
  Brock
  bulldog
  Calman carotid artery
  Calman ring
  Castaneda anastomosis
  Castaneda vascular
  celiac
  coarctation
  Cooley anastomosis
  Cooley aortic
  Cooley coarctation
  Cooley iliac
  Cooley partial occlusion
  Cooley patent ductus
  Cooley pediatric
  Cooley renal
  Cooley vascular
  Cooley vena cava catheter
  Cooley-Beck
  Cooley-Derra anastomosis
  Cooley-Satinsky

clamp *(cont.)*
 Crafoord aortic
 Crafoord coarctation
 curved
 Davidson vessel
 Davis aneurysm
 DeBakey aortic aneurysm
 DeBakey arterial
 DeBakey bulldog
 DeBakey coarctation
 DeBakey cross-action bulldog
 DeBakey patent ductus
 DeBakey pediatric
 DeBakey peripheral vascular
 DeBakey ring-handled bulldog
 DeBakey tangential occlusion
 DeBakey vascular
 DeBakey-Bahnson vascular
 DeBakey-Bainbridge
 DeBakey-Beck
 DeBakey-Derra anastomosis
 DeBakey-Harken
 DeBakey-Howard
 DeBakey-Kay
 DeBakey-Reynolds anastomosis
 DeBakey-Semb
 DeMartel vascular
 Demos tibial artery
 DeWeese vena cava
 exclusion
 Fogarty-Chin
 Fogarty Hydrogrip
 Garcia aorta clamp
 Gerbode patent ductus
 Glover coarctation
 Glover patent ductus
 Glover vascular
 Grant aneurysm
 Gregory baby profunda clamp
 Gregory carotid bulldog
 Gregory external
 Gross coarctation occlusion
 Grover
 Gutgeman
 Harken auricle

clamp *(cont.)*
 Heifitz
 hemostatic
 Hendrin ductus
 Henley vascular
 Hopkins aortic
 Hufnagel aortic
 Humphries aortic
 Jacobson-Potts
 Jahnke anastomosis
 Javid carotid artery
 Johns Hopkins coarctation
 Jones thoracic
 Kapp-Beck
 Kapp-Beck-Thomson
 Kartchner carotid artery
 Kay aorta
 Kay-Lambert
 Kindt carotid artery
 Lambert aortic
 Lambert-Kay aorta
 Lambert-Kay vascular
 Lee microvascular
 Leland-Jones vascular
 Liddle aorta
 Mason vascular
 Mattox aorta
 metal
 metallic
 Michel aortic
 Mixter right-angle
 Morris aorta
 mosquito
 Muller pediatric
 Niedner anastomosis
 noncrushing vascular
 Noon AV fistula
 occluding
 O'Neill
 partial occlusion
 partially occluding vascular
 patent ductus
 Pean
 pediatric bulldog
 pediatric vascular

clamp *(cont.)*
   Poppen-Blalock-Salibi
   Potts aortic
   Potts coarctation
   Potts patent ductus
   Potts-Nieder
   Potts-Satinsky
   Potts-Smith aortic occlusion
   Reinhoff
   Reynolds vascular
   right-angle
   Rumel myocardial
   Rumel thoracic
   Salibi carotid artery
   Sarot bronchus
   Satinsky aortic
   Satinsky vascular
   Satinsky vena cava
   Schmidt
   Schumaker aortic
   Schwartz
   Sehrt
   Selman
   Selverstone carotid
   side-biting
   sponge
   spoon
   stainless steel
   Stille-Crawford
   straight
   Subramanian
   Swan aortic
   Thompson carotid artery
   tissue occlusion
   tube-occluding
   tubing
   vascular
   Vorse-Webster
   Wangensteen anastomosis
   Wangensteen patent ductus
   Weber aortic
   Wister vascular
   Wylie carotid artery
   Yasargil carotid
Clark oxygen electrode
classification
   American Heart Association (AHA) stenosis
   Cedars-Sinai pump failure
   Dexter-Grossman mitral regurgitation
   Fredrickson hyperlipoproteinemia
   Killip heart disease
   Killip pump failure
   Killip-Kimball heart failure
   Lev complete AV block
   Levine-Harvey heart murmur
   Lown ventricular arrhythmia
   Lown ventricular premature beat
   Minnesota EKG
   NYHA (New York Heart Association) congestive heart failure
   NYHA angina
   TIMI (thrombolysis in myocardial infarction)
   Vaughn Williams antiarrhythmic drugs
Classix pacemaker
claudication
   buttock
   calf
   hip
   intermittent
   leg
   lifestyle-limiting
   lower extremity
   nonlifestyle-limiting
   one-block
   thigh
   three-block
   two-block
   two-flights-of-stairs
   venous
cleft
   cholesterol
   Sondergaard
click
   aortic
   aortic ejection

click *(cont.)*
   ejection
   loud
   midsystolic
   nonejection systolic (NESC)
   pulmonary ejection
   systolic
   systolic ejection
   systolic nonejection
   valvular
clinometry
clip (see *clamp*)
Clip On torquer
clockwise rotation of electrical axis on EKG
closure
   patch
   primary
   secondary
   valve
clot formation
clots and debris
Cloverleaf catheter
clubbing of fingernails; fingertips
clubbing of fingers and toes
clubbing, cyanosis, or edema (C, C, or E)
CM_5 lead
CMR (congenital mitral regurgitation)
CMT (circus-movement tachycardia)
CO (cardiac output) (L/min)
CO_2 laser
Co-A reductase
coagulation, disseminated intravascular (DIC)
coagulator
   Biceps bipolar
   Concept bipolar
Coanda effect
coaptation of valve leaflets
coarctation of aorta
   postductal
   preductal
   reversed

coarctectomy
Cobe-Stockert heart-lung machine
Cobra catheter
Code Blue
codominant coronary circulation
codominant vessel
coeur en sabot (on x-ray)
coil, Gianturco wool-tufted wire
coil-tipped catheter
cold potassium cardioplegia
cold pressor stimulation
cold pressor test (Hines and Brown test)
coldness of extremity
Cole-Cecil murmur
collagen vascular screen (test)
collateral, collaterals
   antegrade
   arcade of
   bridging
   filled by
   filling via
   gives
   left to left
   persistent congenital stenosed
   receives
   retrograde
   right to left
   septal
collateral circulation
collateral vessel filling
collateralization, distal
Collins bicycle ergometer
Collostat hemostatic sponge
columnae carneae
Comfeel Ulcus dressing
Command PS pacemaker
commissure
   fused
   scalloped
   valve
commissurotomy
   Brockenbrough transseptal
   closed
   closed mitral

commissurotomy *(cont.)*
   mitral valve
   open mitral
   percutaneous catheter
   percutaneous transvenous mitral (PTMC)
commode, bedside
Commucor A+V Patient Monitor
communicators, stripping of multiple
comp (comparison)
compartment syndrome
compensated congestive heart failure
compensated edentulism (false teeth)
compensatory mechanism
compensatory pause
competent valve
complete atrioventricular block
complete atrioventricular dissociation
complex
   aberrant QRS
   anomalous
   atrial
   AV junctional escape
   biphasic EKG
   diphasic EKG
   Eisenmenger
   frequent spontaneous premature
   fusion QRS
   interpolated premature
   Lutembacher
   monophasic contour of QRS
   multiform premature ventricular
   normal-voltage QRS
   parasystolic ventricular
   preexcited QRS
   premature atrial (PAC)
   premature AV junctional
   premature ventricular
   QRS
   QRS-T
   RS
   slurring of QRS

complex *(cont.)*
   triphasic contour of QRS
   ventricular
   ventricular escape
   ventricular premature (VPC)
   wide QRS
   widening of QRS
complex ventricular ectopic activity
compliance, ventricular
composite valve graft replacement
compression stockings, Sigvaris
compromise, systemic circulatory
Compuscan Hittman computerized electrocardioscanner
Concato disease
concentric left ventricular hypertrophy
Concept bipolar coagulator
conduction
   aberrant
   accelerated AV node
   anomalous
   antegrade
   anterograde
   concealed
   decremental
   delayed
   infranodal
   intra-atrial
   intraventricular
   preexcitation
   retrograde
   retrograde VA
   supernormal
   ventriculoatrial (VA)
conduction defect
conduction delay
conduction disturbance
conduction ratio (number of P waves to number of QRS)
conduction system
conduit (see *graft*)
congenital heart failure (CHF)
congestion, pulmonary venous

connection
   partial anomalous pulmonary
      venous
   total anomalous pulmonary
      venous (TAPVC)
conotruncal anomaly, congenital
Conray contrast medium
consent, written informed
constrictive pericarditis
consumption
   myocardial oxygen (MVO_2)
   ventilatory oxygen (VO_2)
continuity equation
continuous ambulatory peritoneal
   dialysis
contractile pattern
contractile work index
contractility
   cardiac
   myocardial
contractility index
contraction
   atrial premature (APC)
   automatic ventricular
   cardiac
   escaped ventricular
   isovolumelic (IVC)
   nodal premature
   premature atrial (PAC)
   premature junctional (PJC)
   premature nodal (PNC)
   premature ventricular (PVC)
   R-on-T ventricular premature
   supraventricular premature
      (SVPC)
   ventricular premature (VPC)
   ventricular segmental
contractor
   Bailey rib
   Bailey-Gibbon rib
   rib
contralateral vessel
contrast medium; media
   (see also *dye*)
   Amipaque

contrast medium *(cont.)*
   Angio-Conray
   Angiocontrast
   Angiovist 282; 292; 370
   carbonated saline solution
   Conray
   Conray-30; -43; -400
   degassed tap water
   dextrose 5% in water
   diatrizoate meglumine
   diatrizoate sodium
   Diatrizoate-60
   hand-agitated
   Hexabrix
   hydrogen peroxide
   Hypaque Meglumine
   Hypaque Sodium
   Hypaque-76; -M
   indocyanine green
   iohexol
   iopamidol
   Iopamiron 310; 370
   iothalamate meglumine
   iothalamate sodium
   ioxaglate meglumine
   Isovue-300; -370, Isovue-M 300
   mannitol and saline 1:1 solution
   MD-60; MD-76
   Omnipaque
   polygelin colloid
   Renografin-60; -76
   Renovist
   Renovist II
   SHU-454
   sodium bicarbonate solution
   sodium chloride 0.9%
   sonicated meglumine sodium
   sonicated Renografin-76
   sorbitol 70%
   Thorotrast
   Ultravist
   Urografin-76
   Vascoray
   ZK44012
contusion, myocardial

conus artery; ligament
conus arteriosus
conversion, spontaneous
convexo-concave disk prosthetic valve
Cook arterial catheter
Cook deflector
Cook pacemaker
Cook yellow pigtail catheter
Cooley anastomosis clamp
Cooley aortic clamp
Cooley atrial retractor
Cooley coarctation clamp
Cooley iliac clamp
Cooley intrapericardial anastomosis
Cooley modification of Waterston anastomosis
Cooley partial occlusion clamp
Cooley patent ductus clamp
Cooley pediatric clamp
Cooley renal clamp
Cooley retractor
Cooley valve dilator
Cooley vascular clamp
Cooley vascular forceps
Cooley vena cava catheter clamp
Cooley-Baumgarten aortic forceps
Cooley-Beck clamp
Cooley-Cutter disk prosthetic valve
Cooley-Derra anastomosis clamp
Cooley-Satinsky clamp
cooling, core
Coombs murmur
Coombs test
  direct
  indirect
Cooper ligament
COPD (chronic obstructive pulmonary disease)
Cope biopsy needle
Cope needle introducer cannula
cor (heart)
cor adiposum
cor arteriosum
cor biloculare

cor bovinum
cor dextrum
cor hirsutum
cor pendulum
cor pseudotriloculare biatriatum
cor pulmonale
cor sinistrum
cor taurinum
cor triatriatum
cor triloculare
cor triloculare biatriatum
cor triloculare biventriculare
cor venosum
cor villosum
Coratomic prosthetic valve
Cordis Brite Tip guiding catheter
Cordis-Ducor-Judkins
Cordis electrode
Cordis Gemini pacemaker
Cordis high flow pigtail catheter
Cordis lead conversion kit
Cordis Multicor II pacemaker
Cordis pacing lead
Cordis Sequicor II pacemaker
Cordis sheath
core cooling
core of atheroma
core temperature
Cormed pump
corneal arcus
Corometrics-Aloka echocardiograph machine
coronary arteriography
coronary artery bypass graft (CABG)
coronary artery dominance
coronary artery lesion
coronary artery malformation
coronary blood flow, regional
coronary bypass graft patency
coronary care unit (CCU)
coronary cusp
coronary disease, three-vessel
coronary flow reserve (CFR)
coronary ostium

coronary sclerosis
coronary sinus (CS)
coronary sinus rhythm (CSR)
coronary steal phenomenon
coronary steal syndrome
COROSKOP C cardiac imaging system
corrected sinus node recovery time (CSNRT)
corrected transposition of great arteries (CTGA)
Corrigan disease
Corrigan pulse
Corrigan sign
Corvisart disease
Cosmos pulse generator pacemaker
Cosmos 283 DDD pacemaker
Cosmos II DDD pacemaker
Cosmos pulse generator
costoclavicular maneuver
costophrenic angle
CO_2 laser
cottage loaf appearance (on x-ray)
cough, decubitus
cough-thrill
Coulter counter for platelet count
coumadinization
count
   complete blood cell (CBC)
   needle, sponge, and instrument
   platelet
   RBC (red blood cell)
   reticulocyte
   WBC (white blood cell)
counterpulsation
   intra-aortic balloon
   percutaneous intra-aortic balloon (PIBC)
countershock, unsynchronized
couplet, ventricular
coupling interval
Cournand catheter; needle
course of the vessel
coved ST segments
coxsackievirus

CPAD (chronic peripheral arterial disease)
CPAP (continuous positive airway pressure)
CPB (cardiopulmonary bypass)
CPI (Cardiac Pacemakers, Inc.) pacemaker
CPI Astra pacemaker
CPI automatic implantable defibrillator
CPI L67 electrode
CPI 910 ULTRA II pacemaker
CPI porous tined-tip bipolar pacing lead
CPI Sweet Tip lead
CPK (creatine phosphokinase)
CPK isoenzymes: CPK-MB; CPK-MM
CPK, MB positive
CPR (cardiopulmonary resuscitation), closed chest
cps (cycles per second)
Crafoord aortic clamp
Crafoord coarctation clamp
Crafoord thoracic scissors
cramps, calf
Crampton test
cranial and caudal angulations
cranial angulation, anteroposterior x-ray projection with
cranial view
crash induction of anesthesia
Crawford aortic retractor
Crawford suture ring
Crawford technique for thoracoabdominal aneurysm
Crawford-Cooley tunneler
crease, earlobe
creatine kinase (CK) isoenzymes
   CK-BB (CK_1)
   CK-MB (CK_2)
   CK-MM (CK_3)
creatine phosphokinase (CPK)
creatinine
crescendo angina; murmur

crescendo-decrescendo murmur
crest
　infundibuloventricular
　supraventricular
CREST syndrome
CRF (chronic renal failure; chronic reserve flow)
Crile forceps
Crile hemostat
crimp, crimper, crimping
crisis, hypertensive
crisscross fashion; heart
crista supraventricularis
crista terminalis
critical care unit (CCU)
Critikon catheter
cross-clamp (noun)
cross-clamped (verb)
cross-clamping of aorta
Cross-Jones disk prosthetic valve
cross-pelvic collateral vessel
crossover femoral-femoral bypass
crosstalk
CRS (catheter-related sepsis)
Crump vessel dilator
crunch, Hamman
crushing chest pain
Cruveilhier-Baumgarten murmur
crux
crux cordis (crux of heart)
crux dextrum fasciculi atrioventricularis
crux sinistrum fasciculi atrioventricularis
cryoablation catheter
cryoablation, encircling endocardial
cryopreserved allograft
cryopreserved homograft tissue
cryopreserved human allograft conduit
cryopreserved human aortic allograft
cryosurgery, map-guided
crystalloid
crystalloid cardioplegic solution
crystalloid prime for heart-lung machine
CS (coronary sinus)
CSA (cross-sectional area)
CSH (carotid sinus hypersensitivity)
CSI (coronary stenosis index)
CSICU (cardiac surgery intensive care unit)
CSNRT (corrected sinus node recovery time)
CSR (coronary sinus rhythm)
CSS (carotid sinus syndrome)
CT scan, ultrafast
CTGA (corrected transposition of great arteries)
CTR (cardiothoracic ratio; cardiac transplant recipient)
cuff
　aortic
　atrial
　blood pressure
　pneumatic
　right atrial
current of injury
curve
　AA
　A_1A_2
　AH
　A_2H_2
　arterial dilution
　ascorbate dilution
　central intra-aortic pressure
　dye
　indicator dilution
　indicator dye-dilution
　indocyanine dilution
　intracardiac dye-dilution
　left ventricular inflow velocity
　oxyhemoglobin dissociation
　time activity (for contrast agent)
　V_2A_2
　V_1V_2
　venous dilution
　ventricular function
curvilinear aortotomy

Cushing forceps
Cushing reflex
Cushing rongeur
Cushing vein retractor
cushion, endocardial
cusp
   accessory
   aortic
   asymmetric closure of
   conjoined
   coronary
   cuspid
   dysplastic
   fish-mouth
   fusion of
   noncoronary
   septic perforation of
   valve
cusp degenerator
cusp fenestration
cusp motion
cusp shots (films)
cuspis anterior valvae atrioventricularis dextrae
cuspis anterior valvae atrioventricularis sinistrae
cuspis posterior valvae atrioventricularis dextrae
cuspis posterior valvae atrioventricularis sinistrae
cuspis septalis valvae atrioventricularis dextrae
cut and cine film
cutdown (noun)
   brachial
   femoral
cutis marmorata
cutter
   atherectomy
   Leather valve
   wire
Cutter aortic valve prosthesis

Cutter-Smeloff cardiac valve prosthesis
Cutter-Smeloff heart valve
cutting device
CV wave of jugular venous pulse
CVA (cerebrovascular accident) (stroke)
CVA, posterior circulation
CVC (central venous catheterization)
CVIS imaging device
CVP (central venous pressure) catheter
CVRI (coronary vascular resistance index)
CXR (chest x-ray), baseline
cyanosis
   central
   circumoral
   mucous membrane
   peripheral
   shunt
   systemic
   tardive pulmonary
cyanosis, clubbing, or edema (C, C, or E)
cyanosis of nail beds
Cyberlith multiprogrammable pulse generator
Cyberlith pacemaker
Cybertach 60 pacemaker
Cybertach automatic-burst atrial pacemaker
cycle
   cardiac
   length of atrial
   length of ventricular
   RR
   sinus length (SLC)
cycle-ergometer
cycles per second (cps)
cyst, pericardial

D

D point; D wave
D1 (diagonal branch #1)
D₅W, D5W, D-5-W (5% dextrose in water)
DaCosta syndrome
Dacron, preclotted tightly woven graft
Dacron catheter
Dacron conduit
Dacron mesh
Dacron onlay patch-graft
Dacron Sauvage patch
Dacron stent
Dacron suture
Dacron tape
Dacron tube graft
Daig ESI-II or DSI-III screw-in lead pacemaker
Dakin Biograft
Dale forceps
dam, left ventricular
damped (adj.); damping (noun)
Dardik Biograft
Datascope System 90 balloon pump
DataVue calibrated reference circle
Davidson scapular retractor
Davidson thoracic trocar
Davidson vessel clamp
Davies endomyocardial fibrosis
Davis aneurysm clip
Davis forceps
Davis rib spreader
Davol pacemaker introducer
DBP (diastolic blood pressure)
DC (direct current) cardioversion
DC defibrillator
DC electrical shock
DCM (dilated cardiomyopathy)
DCS (distal coronary sinus)
dD/dt (derived value on apex cardiogram)
DDD mode

DDD pacemaker
D-E amplitude of mitral valve
D to E slope on echocardiography
deaired graft
deairing maneuver
death
   aborted sudden cardiac (ASCD)
   sudden
   sudden cardiac
Deaver retractor
DeBakey aortic aneurysm clamp
DeBakey arterial clamp; forceps
DeBakey Autaugrip forceps
DeBakey ball valve prosthesis
DeBakey bulldog clamp
DeBakey coarctation clamp
DeBakey cross-action bulldog clamp
DeBakey dissecting forceps
DeBakey endarterectomy scissors
DeBakey patent ductus clamp
DeBakey pediatric clamp
DeBakey peripheral vascular clamp
DeBakey rib spreader
DeBakey ring-handled bulldog clamp
DeBakey tangential occlusion clamp
DeBakey technique for thoraco-abdominal aneurysm
DeBakey tissue forceps
DeBakey valve scissors
DeBakey vascular clamp; forceps
DeBakey-Bahnson vascular clamp
DeBakey-Bainbridge clamp
DeBakey-Beck clamp
DeBakey-Cooley retractor
DeBakey-Derra anastomosis clamp
DeBakey-Diethrich vascular forceps
DeBakey-Harken clamp
DeBakey-Howard clamp
DeBakey-Kay clamp
DeBakey-Reynolds anastomosis clamp

DeBakey-Semb clamp; forceps
DeBakey-Surgitool prosthetic valve
debris
  atheromatous
  calcium
  gelatinous
debubbling procedure
decannulated, decannulation
decompensated congestive heart
  failure
decompensation
  cardiac
  hemodynamic
decompress
decompression of ventricle
decremental element
decubitus cough
deep Doppler velocity interrogation
deep tendon reflex (DTR)
deep venous thrombosis (DVT)
defect
  acquired ventricular septal
    (AVSD)
  aortic septal
  aorticopulmonary septal
  atrial ostium primum
  atrial septal or atrioseptal (ASD)
  atrioventricular canal
  atrioventricular septal
  AV conduction
  conduction
  contiguous ventricular septal
  endocardial cushion
  filling
  fixed perfusion
  inferoapical
  infundibular ventricular septal
  interatrial septum
  interventricular conduction
  interventricular septal (IVSD)
  intra-atrial conduction
  intraluminal filling
  intraventricular conduction
  linear
  luminal

defect *(cont.)*
  membranous ventricular septal
  muscular ventricular septal
  ostium primum
  ostium secundum
  partial AV canal
  perfusion
  peri-infarction conduction
    (PICD)
  postinfarction ventriculoseptal
  reversible ischemic
  reversible perfusion
  scintigraphic perfusion
  secundum and sinus venosus
  secundum atrial septal
  secundum-type atrial septal
  septal
  supracristal ventriculoseptal
  transcatheter closure of atrial
  transient perfusion
  septal
  transient perfusion
  ventriculoseptal (VSD)
defibrillation, single pulse
defibrillator
  AICD-B cardioverter
  AICD-BR cardioverter
  AID-B
  automatic external (AED)
  automatic implantable (or internal) cardioverter (AICD)
  automatic implantable (or internal) (AID)
  CPI automatic implantable
  DC (direct current)
  external cardioverter
  Heart Aid 80
  Hewlett-Packard
  implantable
  Intec implantable
  ODAM
defibrillator unit
deficit
  peripheral pulse
  pulse

deficit *(cont.)*
    reversible intermittent or ischemic neurologic (RIND)
    transient neurological
deflection
    delta
    intrinsicoid
    QS
    RS
deflector, Cook
deformity
    gooseneck outflow tract
    hockey-stick tricuspid valve
    parachute mitral valve
    parachute-type
degeneration
    cardiomyopathic
    cusp
    glassy
    myocardial cellular
degrees of heart block
Dehio test
dehisced, dehiscence
Deklene suture
de Lange syndrome
Delbet sign
Delrin frame of valve prosthesis, Dacron-covered
delta deflection
Delta pacemaker
delta wave
deltopectoral groove
demand mode of pacemaker
demand pacemaker battery
demand pulse generator unit
DeMartel vascular clamp; scissors
Demos tibial artery clamp
de Musset sign
denude, denuding
dep (depressed)
depolarization
    atrial
    cardiac
    His bundle—distal coronary sinus atrial (H-DCSA)

depolarization *(cont.)*
    His bundle—middle coronary sinus atrial (H-MCSA)
    rapid
    ventricular
depression
    downhill ST segment
    horizontal ST segment
    marked ST segment
    reciprocal
    ST segment
Dermalene suture
Dermalon suture
Derra commissurotomy knife
Derra valve dilator
descent
    x
    y
Deseret angiocatheter
Desilets introducer system
Desilets-Hoffman catheter introducer
De Vega annuloplasty
De Vega prosthesis
deviation on EKG
    left axis (LAD)
    right axis (RAD)
device
    abdominal aortic counterpulsation (AACD)
    abdominal left ventricular assist (ALVAD)
    cutting
    CVIS imaging
    Dinamap automated blood pressure
    Doppler
    Hershey left ventricular assist
    intra-aortic balloon assist
    left ventricular assist (LVAD)
    MediPort implantable vascular access
    Novacore left ventricular assist
    PET balloon atherectomy, Simpson

device *(cont.)*
   pulsatile assist (PAD)
   right ventricular assist (RVAD)
   rotational atherectomy
   Symbion pneumatic assist
   Thoratec BVAD (biventricular assist device)
   Thoratec RVAD (right ventricular assist device)
   Thoratec VAD (ventricular assist device)
   ventricular assist (VAD)
   Wizard disposable inflation
Devices, Ltd. pacemaker
devitalized tissue
DeWeese vena cava clip
Dexon suture
Dexter-Grossman classification of mitral regurgitation
Dextran 40; 75
dextran
   high molecular weight
   low molecular weight
dextrocardia, mirror image
dextrorotatory
dextrotransposition (D-transposition) of great arteries
dextroversion of heart
DFP (diastolic filling pressure)
DFT (defibrillation threshold)
diagnostic ST segment changes
diagonal branch
dialysis, continuous ambulatory peritoneal (CAPD)
diameter
   aortic (AD)
   aortic root
   artery
   left anterior internal (LAID)
   left ventricular internal (LVID)
   luminal
   right ventricular internal (RVID)
   stenosis
   transverse cardiac
   valve

diamond-shaped murmur
diaphoresis, diaphoretic
diaphragm of stethoscope
diaphragmatic pericardium
Diasonics transducer
diastole, early
diastolic filling period
diastolic pressure-time index (DPTI)
diastolic regurgitant velocity
diastolic thrill
diatrizoate meglumine contrast medium
diatrizoate sodium contrast medium
Diatrizoate-60 contrast medium
DIC (disseminated intravascular coagulation)
Dick valve dilator
dicrotic notch or wave of carotid arterial pulse
diet
   anticoronary
   Kempner
   low cholesterol
   low in saturated fat
   low salt
   low sodium
   no added salt
   salt-restricted
Diethrich coronary artery instruments
difference
   AV (arteriovenous)
   AVD O_2
   pulmonary AV
   resting AV
   systemic AV
diffuse, diffusion
diffuse ST-T depression
dig (digitalis) level; effect
DiGeorge syndrome
digital runoff
digital subtraction angiography (DSA)
digital videoangiography

digitalis effect; level
digitalis intoxication
digitalis toxicity
digitalize, digitalized
digitalizing dose
digitoxicity
Digitron
dilatation
   aneurysmal
   annular
   idiopathic pulmonary artery
   idiopathic right atrial
   left ventricular
   percutaneous transluminal balloon (PTBD)
   poststenotic
   poststenotic aortic
   right ventricular
   sequential
   ventricular
dilatation of aorta
dilatation of aortic root
dilatation of pulmonary artery
dilatation of ventricular wall
dilation, percutaneous balloon
dilator
   aortic
   Brock cardiac
   Cooley valve
   Crump vessel
   Derra valve
   Dick valve
   Garrett vascular
   Gerbode valve
   Hegar
   Henley
   Hiebert vascular
   Hohn vessel
   Lucchese mitral valve
   mitral valve
   myocardial
   Tubbs mitral valve
   valve
   vein
dilator-sheath

dimension
   aortic root
   left atrial
   left ventricular end-diastolic (LVEDD)
   left ventricular end-systolic (LVESD)
   left ventricular internal diastolic (LVIDD)
   left ventricular internal end-diastole (LVIDd)
   left ventricular internal end-systole (LVIDs)
   left ventricular internal (LVID)
   left ventricular systolic (LVs)
   right ventricular (RVD)
Dinamap automated blood pressure device
Dinamap monitor
Dinamap ultrasound blood pressure manometer
diode, Zener
dip phenomenon
dip, septal
diphasic complex on EKG
diphasic P wave
diphasic T wave
Diplos M pacemaker
dipyridamole echocardiography test
dipyridamole handgrip test
dipyridamole infusion test
dipyridamole thallium-201 scintigraphy
dipyridamole thallium scan
dipyridamole thallium ventriculography
disease
   acquired heart
   Adams-Stokes
   alcoholic heart muscle
   amyloid heart
   aortic valve
   aortic valvular (AVD)
   aortoiliac obstructive valvular
   aortoiliac occlusive

disease *(cont.)*
  aortoiliac vascular
  arteriosclerotic cardiovascular (ASCVD)
  arteriosclerotic heart (ASHD)
  arteriosclerotic peripheral vascular
  asymptomatic left main (ALMD)
  atherosclerotic pulmonary vascular (ASPVD)
  Bannister
  Beau
  Bornholm
  Bouillaud
  Bouveret
  branch
  Buerger
  Buerger-Gruetz
  carcinoid heart
  cardiovascular
  carotid occlusive
  carotid vascular
  Chagas
  Christmas (hemophilia B)
  chronic hypertensive
  chronic obstructive pulmonary (COPD)
  chronic peripheral arterial (CPAD)
  Concato
  congenital heart (CHD)
  coronary artery (CAD)
  coronary heart
  Corrigan
  Corvisart
  cyanotic congenital heart
  diffuse
  Döhle (Doehle)
  Duroziez
  eccentric plaque
  end-stage cardiopulmonary
  eosinophilic endomyocardial
  extracranial vascular
  Fallot
  fibrocalcific rheumatic

disease *(cont.)*
  Friedländer (Friedlaender)
  functional cardiovascular
  functional valve
  Gairdner
  global cardiac
  graft occlusive
  Heberden
  Heubner
  Hodgson
  Horton
  Huchard
  hypereosinophilic heart
  hypertensive cardiovascular (HCVD)
  hypertensive heart (HHD)
  iliac atherosclerotic occlusive
  inflammatory aneurysmal
  intrinsic
  ischemic heart
  ischemic myocardial
  Kussmaul-Maier
  latent coronary artery
  latent ischemic heart
  left anterior descending coronary artery
  left main coronary artery
  left main equivalent
  Lenegre
  Lev
  Libman-Sacks
  Loeffler
  Milton
  mitral valve
  Mondor
  Moschcowitz
  moyamoya (cerebrovascular)
  multivessel coronary artery
  necrotizing arterial
  nonatherosclerotic coronary artery
  nonoperable
  occlusive
  occlusive peripheral arterial
  one-vessel coronary artery

disease *(cont.)*
  organic hcart (OHD)
  organic valve
  Owren (Factor V deficiency)
  pericardial
  peripartal heart
  peripheral arterial
  peripheral atherosclerotic
  peripheral vascular (PVD)
  Pick
  primary myocardial
  pulmonary collagen vascular (PCVD)
  pulmonary heart
  pulmonary vascular obstructive
  pulmonary veno-occlusive (PVOD)
  pulseless
  Quincke
  Raynaud
  rhcumatic heart (RHD)
  rheumatic mitral valve
  rheumatic valvular
  right coronary artery
  Roger
  Rokitansky
  Rougnon-Heberden
  scleroderma heart
  single-vessel heart
  sinoatrial
  sinus node
  Stokes-Adams
  symptomatic left main (SLMD)
  Takayasu
  three-vessel coronary artery
  thyrotoxic heart
  triple coronary artery
  triple-vessel
  two-vessel coronary artery
  valvular (VD)
  valvular heart
  vasculo-Behçet
  von Willebrand
  Wenckebach
  Winiwarter-Buerger

disk, Eigon
disk poppet
disobliteration, carotid
disopyramide
displacement, late systolic
dissected free
dissection
  aortic
  blunt
  finger
  intimal
  sharp
  spiral
dissector
  Holinger
  Jannetta
  Lemmon intimal
  Penfield
  sponge
disseminated intravascular coagulation (DIC)
dissociation
  atrioventricular (AVD)
  AV (atrioventricular)
  complete atrioventricular
  electromechanical
  incomplete atrioventricular (IAVD)
  intracavitary pressure-electrogram
  isorhythmic AV
distal circumflex marginal artery
distal coronary sinus (CS)
distensibility, ventricular
distention
  atrial presystolic
  jugular venous (JVD)
  neck vein
distention of neck veins
distress, respiratory
disturbance, cardiac rhythm
diurese, diuresed, diuresis
diuretic, diuretics
  high-ceiling
  loop
  osmotic

diuretic *(cont.)*
 potassium-sparing
 potassium-wasting
 thiazide
diuretic therapy
DLP cardioplegic catheter; needle
DMI (Diagnostic Medical Instruments) analyzer
DMI (diaphragmatic myocardial infarction)
DMPE (^{99m}Tc-bis-dimethylphosphonoethane)
DOC exchange technique
DOC guide wire extension
dock wire; docking wire
Docke murmur
Dodd perforating vein group
Dodge area-length method for ventricular activity; volume
Dodge method for calculating left ventricular volume
Dodge method for ejection fraction
DOE (dyspnea on exertion)
Doehle (Döhle) disease
dome of atrium
dome and dart configuration on cardiac catheterization
dominance
 coronary artery
 mixed
 right ventricular
 shared coronary artery
doming, diastolic
doming of leaflets
doming of valve
donor organ, appropriately sized and matched
donor organ ischemic time
Doppler
 continuous wave
 pulsed
Doppler blood flow detector
Doppler blood pressure
Doppler color flow imaging, transesophageal
Doppler color flow mapping
Doppler coronary catheter
Doppler device
Doppler echocardiography
Doppler flow probe; study
Doppler imaging
Doppler shift
Doppler signal
Doppler study, periorbital
Doppler velocimetry
Doplette
Doptone monitor of fetal heart tones
Dorendorf sign
Dorros brachial internal mammary guiding catheter
dorsalis pedis pulse
dose, tracer
DORV (double outlet right ventricle)
dose
 digitalizing
 loading
Dotter caged balloon catheter
Dotter coaxial catheter
Dotter Intravascular Retrieval Set
Dotter method; system
Dotter-Judkins technique in percutaneous transluminal angioplasty
doughnut configuration on thallium imaging
Douglas bag
Dow method for cardiac output
Down syndrome
downhill ST segment depression
downsloping ST segment depression
downstream sampling method
downward sloping
doxorubicin cardiotoxicity
Doyen rib elevator
Doyen rib rasp; raspatory
dP/dt (upstroke pattern on apex cardiogram)
DPTI (diastolic pressure-time index)
drainage
 closed chest

drainage *(cont.)*
   total anomalous pulmonary venous
dressing
   Comfeel Ulcus
   stent
   Synthaderm
   Vigilon
   wet-to-dry
Dressler syndrome
drip, I.V. (intravenous)
drive cycle length
drug-resistant tachyarrhythmia
Drummond sign
DSA (digital subtraction angiography)
DSAS (discrete subvalvular aortic stenosis)
DTAF-F (descending thoracic aortofemoral-femoral) bypass
DTPA, technetium bound to
DTR (deep tendon reflex)
D-transposition (dextrotransposition) of great arteries
dual-chamber pacemaker
Ducor balloon catheter
Ducor-Cordis pigtail catheter
Ducor HF (high-flow) catheter
ductulus
ductus arteriosus
   patent (PDA)
   persistent
   reversed
ductus venosus
Duffield scissors
Duke bleeding time: test
dullness
   cardiac
   left border of cardiac (LBCD)
   percussion
   tympanitic
Dunlop thrombus stripper
Duostat
duplex Doppler ultrasound
duplex scanning

Duran annuloplasty ring
Durapulse pacemaker
duration, action potential (APD)
duration of EKG wave
duration of exercise
duration of P wave
duration of QRS
Duroziez disease: sign
Duroziez murmur
Duval-Crile lung forceps
DVI Simpson atherocath
DVT (deep venous thrombosis)
dye (see also *contrast medium)*
   Cardio-Green
   Fox green
   indocyanine green
dye curve
dyne
dysbetalipoproteinemia, familial
dyscontrol
dysfunction
   focal ventricular
   global ventricular
   left ventricular (LVD)
   mitral valve (MVD)
   papillary muscle (PMD)
   regional myocardial
   sinus node
   ventricular
dyskinesia, regional
dyskinesis
   anteroapical
   left ventricular
dyskinetic
dysmodulation
dysphagia
dysplasia
   arrhythmogenic right ventricular
   pulmonary valve (PVD)
   ventricular
dysplastic
dyspnea
   cardiac
   exertional
   nocturnal

dyspnea *(cont.)*
  paroxysmal nocturnal (PND)
dyspnea at rest
dyspnea on exertion (DOE)
dyspncic

dysrhythmia
Dysshwannian syndrome
dyssynergia
  regional
  segmental

E

E/A ratio on echocardiogram
E to F slope
E point of cardiac apex pulse
E point on apex cardiogram
E point on echocardiogram
E point to septal separation (EPSS)
E sign (on x-ray)
ear oximetry
earlobe crease (probable risk sign for coronary artery disease)
EBDA (effective balloon dilated area)
EBL (estimated blood loss)
Ebstein anomaly; sign
ECA (external carotid artery)
E-CABG (endarterectomy and coronary artery bypass graft)
eccentric atrial activation
eccentric ledge
eccentric plaque disease
eccentric stenosis
ECG (electrocardiogram)
ECG rhythm strip
ECG-synchronized digital subtraction angiography
echo (echocardiogram)
echocardiogram, -graphy
  akinesis on
  ambulatory Holter
  A-mode
  anterior left ventricular wall motion
  apical
  apical five-chamber view

echocardiogram *(cont.)*
  apical four-chamber view
  apical left ventricular wall motion on
  apical two-chamber view
  B bump on anterior mitral valve leaflet
  cardiac output
  color flow imaging Doppler
  continuous loop exercise
  contrast
  contrast-enhanced
  cross-sectional two-dimensional
  CW (continuous wave) Doppler
  D to E slope on
  Doppler
  dyskinesis on
  E point on
  echo-free space on
  echo intensity disappearance rate on
  exercise
  Feigenbaum
  four-chamber
  hypokinesis on
  inferior left ventricular wall motion on
  intracoronary contrast
  intraoperative cardioplegic contrast
  lateral left ventricular wall motion on
  late systolic posterior displacement on

echocardiogram *(cont.)*
  left ventricular long-axis
  long-axis parasternal view
  loss of an "a" dip on
  Meridian
  M-mode Doppler
  myocardial contrast (MCE)
  myocardial perfusion
  parasternal long-axis view
  parasternal short-axis view
  postcontrast
  posterior left ventricular wall motion on
  postexercise
  postinjection
  postmyocardial
  precontrast
  preinjection
  premyocardial
  pulsed Doppler
  pulsed-wave (PW) Doppler
  real-time
  resting
  right ventricular short-axis
  septal wall motion on
  short-axis view
  signal averaged
  stress
  subcostal short-axis view
  subxiphoid view of
  transesophageal (TEE)
  two-chamber
  two-dimensional (2-D)
  ventricular wall motion
echo, echoes
  amphoric
  atrial
  dense
  linear
  metallic
  ventricular (on EKG)
echo-free space
echo reverberation
echogenic mass
echophonocardiography, combined
  M-mode

Echovar Doppler system
ECS (cardioplegic solution)
ectasia, annuloaortic
ectasia of coronary artery
Ectocor pacemaker
ectopia, cordis
ectopic ventricular beat
ectopy
  asymptomatic complex (ACE)
  atrial
  bursts of ventricular
  high-density ventricular
  supraventricular
  ventricular
ED (emergency department)
eddy sound of patent ductus arteriosus
edema
  acute pulmonary
  ankle
  bland
  brawny
  cardiac
  cardiopulmonary
  dependent
  fingerprint
  high-altitude pulmonary
  idiopathic
  localized
  lymphatic
  nonpitting
  paroxysmal pulmonary
  passive
  pedal
  periorbital
  peripheral
  perivascular
  pitting
  pretibial
  pulmonary
  sacral
  stasis
  trace
  venous
edema, cyanosis, or clubbing
edematous

edentulism, compensated (false teeth)
edge
  leading
  shelving
  trailing
Edmark mitral valve
EDRF (endothelium-relaxing factor)
EDVI (end-diastolic volume index)
Edwards diagnostic catheter
Edwards-Duromedics bi-leaflet valve
EF (ejection fraction)
E to F slope of valve
E to F slope on echocardiogram
effect, potassium-sparing
effective refractory period (ERP)
efficacy of drug therapy
efficacy of treatment
effusion
  cholesterol pericardial
  hemorrhagic
  loculated
  malignant
  pericardial (PE)
  pleural
  serofibrinous pericardial
  subpleural
Ehlers-Danlos syndrome
Eigon disk
Einthoven law for EKG
Einthoven triangle
Eisenmenger complex
Eisenmenger reaction with septal defects
Eisenmenger syndrome
ejection fraction (EF)
  area-length method for
  basilar half
  blunted
  BSA (body surface area)
  digital
  Dodge method for
  global
  interval
  Kennedy method for calculating

ejection fraction *(cont.)*
  left ventricular (LVEF)
  one-third
  regional
  resting left ventricular
  right ventricular (RVEF)
  systolic
  thermodilution
EJV (external jugular vein)
EKG (electrocardiogram)
EKG rhythm strip
Ela pacemaker
elastance, maximum ventricular (E_{MAX})
Elecath thermodilution catheter
electrical axis on EKG, J point
electrical events of the EKG
electrical potential
electrocardiogram (ECG or EKG)
  ambulatory (AECG)
  baseline
  Burdick
  computerized
  Corometrics-Aloka
  esophageal
  evolutionary changes on
  exercise
  fetal
  flat
  flatline
  His bundle
  intracardiac
  intracavitary recording of
  intracoronary
  Micro-Tracer portable
  normal resting
  postconversion
  precordial
  pre-exercise resting supine
  resting
  scalar
  serial changes in
  signal-averaged (SAECG)
  signal-averaging technique
  16-lead

electrocardiogram *(cont.)*
  stress
  surface
  telephone transmission of
  three-channel
  three-lead
  12-lead
  vector
electrocardiophonogram
electrocardioscanner, Compuscan
  Hittman computerized
electrode (see also *lead*)
  Arzco TAPSUL pill
  barbed-hook pacemaker
  Biotronik IE 65-I pacemaker
  bipolar pacemaker
  Bisping design
  catheter
  Clark oxygen
  Cordis
  corkscrew-tip pacemaker
  CPI L67
  CPI porous tine-tipped bipolar pacing
  endocardial pacemaker
  endocardial placement of
  epicardial pacemaker
  epicardial patch
  esophageal pill
  flanged
  flanged Silastic tip pacemaker
  floating
  free end of
  hand-held
  His bundle
  J orthogonal
  J-shaped pacemaker
  Laserdish
  Medtronic pacemaker
  Medtronic bipolar
  multiple point
  myocardial
  negative pacemaker
  negative pacing
  orthogonal

electrode *(cont.)*
  pacemaker's indifferent
  pacing
  paddle
  permanent pacing
  pill
  platinum
  point
  positive pacemaker
  positive pacing
  precordial surface
  quadripolar catheter
  Quinton
  ring tip
  screw-in tip pacemaker
  sensing
  Siemens
  Silastic
  skin
  stainless steel
  stimulating
  subxiphoid
  target tip
  Telectronics pacemaker
  temporary pacemaker
  temporary pacing electrode
  temporary transvenous catheter
  thermistor
  thoracic
  three-turn
  tined
  tine-tipped pacemaker
  transesophageal (TEE)
  transthoracic
  transvenous placement of
  two-turn
  unipolar pacemaker
  urethane
  Waterston pacing
  wire
electrode catheter tip
electrode gel
electrode pads
electrode paste
Electrodyne pacemaker

electrogram
  coronary sinus
  CSos (coronary sinus ostium)
  esophageal
  fractionated ventricular
  His bundle (HBE)
  HRA (high right atrium)
  intra-atrial
  intracardiac
  intracoronary
  right atrial
  RVA (right ventricular apical)
  sinus node
electrolytes, *consisting of:*
  bicarbonate (bicarb; HCO_3)
  calcium (Ca)
  chloride (Cl)
  potassium (K)
  sodium (Na)
electromagnetic interference (EMI)
electromechanical dissociation
electrophoresis
electrophysiologic mapping
electrophysiologic study (EPS)
electrovectorcardiogram, -graphy
Elema-Schonander pacemaker
elephant on chest, feeling of
elev (elevated)
elevated gradient
elevation of enzymes
elevation pallor of extremity
elevation
  ST segment
  transient ST segment
elevator
  Doyen rib
  Freer
  Matson rib
  Matson-Alexander rib
  Penfield
  rib
elfin facies
El Gamal coronary bypass catheter
Elgiloy frame of prosthetic valve
Ellestad treadmill exercise protocol

Ellis-van Creveld syndrome
E$_{MAX}$ (ventricular elastance, maximum)
embarrassment, circulatory
embolectomy
  arterial
  pulmonary
embolic event
embolic phenomenon
embolic shower
embolism
  air
  arterial
  capillary
  catheter
  coronary
  direct
  fat
  multiple
  paradoxical
  plasmodium
  pulmonary
  venous
embolization, Silastic bead
embolotherapy, catheter
embolus, emboli
  catheter-induced
  coronary artery
  intraluminal
  paradoxical
  polyurethane foam
  prosthetic valve
  pulmonary (PE)
  saddle
EMD (electromechanical dissociation) of the heart
emergent, emergently
Emerson vein stripper
EMF (endomyocardial fibrosis)
EMI (electromagnetic interference)
EMI-induced pacemaker failure
en bloc
encephalopathy, hypertensive
Encor pacemaker
end diastole

endarterectomy
  aortoiliac
  aortoiliofemoral
  carotid bifurcation
  carotid eversion
  coronary
  gas
  innominate
  laser
  manual core
  profunda
  subclavian
endarterectomy and coronary artery bypass graft (E-CABG)
end-diastolic pressure
end-diastolic volume
endocardial catheter ablation
endocardial cushion
endocardial mapping
endocardial-to-epicardial resection
endocardiectomy
endocarditis
  acute bacterial (ABE)
  acute infective
  aortic valve
  atypical verrucous
  bacterial
  chronic
  constrictive
  enterococcal
  fungal
  gonococcal
  infectious
  infective
  Libman-Sacks
  Loeffler parietal fibroplastic
  malignant
  marantic
  mural
  mycotic
  nonbacterial thrombotic (NBTE)
  nonbacterial verrucous
  parietal
  parietal fibroplastic

endocarditis *(cont.)*
  postoperative
  prosthetic valve
  pulmonic
  rheumatic
  rickettsial
  right-side
  septic
  staphylococcal
  streptococcal
  subacute bacterial (SBE)
  subacute infective
  syphilitic
  thrombotic
  tricuspid valve
  tuberculous
  ulcerative
  valvular
  vegetative
  verrucous
  viridans
endocarditis benigna
endocarditis chordalis
endocarditis lenta
endocardium
endoluminal stent
endomyocardial biopsy
Endotak-C lead
endothelialization of vascular graft
endotracheal tube
Endotrol tracheal tube
endovascular
endpoint, exercise
end-stage cardiomyopathy
end-stage cardiopulmonary disease
end-stage congestive heart failure
end-stage renal disease
end systole
end-systolic volume
Enertrax pacemaker
Enhanced Torque 8F guiding catheter
enlargement (see *hypertrophy*)
entrainment, transient

entrapment, popliteal artery
enucleated
enzyme study
enzymes (see also *isoenzymes*)
   cardiac
   elevated
   myocardial
EP (electrophysiology) study
EPBF (effective pulmonary blood flow)
epicardial attachment
epicardial Doppler flow transducer
epicardial fat tag
epicardial pacemaker electrode
epicardial patch cathode
epicardial reflection
epicardial space
epicardial surface
epicarditis
Eppendorf catheter
EPS (electrophysiologic study)
EPSS (E point to septal separation)
EPTFE (expanded polytetrafluoroethylene) vascular suture
equation
   Bernoulli
   Carter
   continuity
   Hagenbach extension of Poiseuille
   Krovetz and Gessner
   Teichholz
equivocal exercise test
ER (emergency room)
Erb area
Erb point (of heart)
ergometer
   arm
   bicycle
   Bosch ERG 500
   Collins bicycle
   Siemens-Albis bicycle
ergonovine infusion; test

ERP (effective refractory period)
   atrial
   ventricular
erythema marginatum
erythema migrans
erythrocyte sedimentation rate (ESR)
escape beat
Esmarch bandage
esophageal angina
esophageal electrocardiogram
esophageal temperature
ESP (end-systolic pressure)
ESP/ESV ratio
ESR (erythrocyte sedimentation rate)
EST (extrastimulus testing)
Estes EKG criteria/score
estimated blood loss (EBL)
ESV (end-systolic volume)
ESVI (end-systolic volume index)
ESWI/ESVI (end-systolic wall stress index/end-systolic volume index)
ET (ejection time)
Ethibond suture
Ethicon suture
Ethiflex suture
Ethilon suture
etiology
ETT (exercise tolerance test)
eukinesis
eustachian valve
euvolemic
eventration (peaking)
evolution of EKG
evolutionary changes on EKG
Ewart sign
exacerbation of chronic congestive heart failure
examination
   cardiac
   lower extremity
   peripheral vascular
Excimer (from "excited dimer") laser

excrescence, Lambl
excursion, decreased valve
exercise
  active
  active assisted
  active resistive
  isometric
  isometric handgrip
  isotonic
  peak
  rehabilitation
  submaximal
  symptom-limited
exercise capacity
exercise duration (in minutes)
exercise electrocardiography
exercise endpoint
exercise-induced myocardial
  ischemia
exercise load (kpm/min)
exercise stress test, positive
exercise thallium-201 stress test
exercise tolerance, decreased
exercise tolerance test (ETT), graded
exertion, pain precipitated by
exertional angina
exposure to cold, pain precipitated by
exsanguinate(d)

extended collection device
external carotid steal syndrome
extirpation of valve
extracardiac conduit
extracorporeal circulation
extraction, O_2
extrastimulation
extrastimulus, extrastimuli
  critically timed
  double
  paired
  premature
  single
  triple
extrastimulus technique
extrastimulus testing (EST)
extrasystole
  atrial
  atrioventricular
  infranodal
  interpolated
  nodal
  nonpropagated junctional
  premature ventricular
  retrograde
  ventricular
exudate
  fibrinous
  retinal

F

F point of cardiac apex pulse
f wave of jugular venous pulse
F-18 2-deoxyglucose uptake on PET scan
FiO_2 (forced inspiratory oxygen)
Fab fragment, antimyosin
factor, blood coagulation
  AcG (accelerator globulin)
  I: fibrinogen
  II: prothrombin
  III: thromboplastin

factor, blood coagulation *(cont.)*
  IV: calcium ions
  V: proaccelerin (or AcG, accelerator globulin)
  VII: proconvertin (or SPCA, serum prothrombin conversion accelerator)
  VIII: antihemophilic (von Willebrand)
  IX: plasma thromboplastin component (Christmas)

factor, blood coagulation *(cont.)*
   X: Stuart (or Stuart-Prower)
   XI: plasma thromboplastin antecedent
   XII: Hageman
   XIII: fibrin stabilizing
factor
   antihemophilic blood coagulation
   atrial natriuretic (ANF)
   Christmas blood coagulation
   endothelium-relaxing (EDRF)
   rheumatoid arthritis
   von Willebrand blood coagulation
FAI (functional aerobic impairment)
failure
   acute heart
   biventricular heart
   chronic renal
   compensated congestive heart
   congestive heart (CHF)
   decompensated congestive heart
   end-stage congestive heart
   heart
   high-output cardiac
   left-sided congestive heart
   left ventricular
   primary bioprosthetic valve
   pump
   refractory congestive heart
   respiratory
   right heart
   right ventricular
   right-sided congestive heart
Fallot disease
Fallot pentalogy (tetralogy of Fallot plus atrial septal defect)
Fallot tetralogy, pink
family history of heart disease
family history of myocardial infarction
Family Index of Life Events (FILE)
FAP (femoral artery pressure)
fascia, fasciae
   pectoralis
   prepectoral

fascicle
   left anterior
   left posterior
fascicular heart block
fasciculoventricular bypass fiber; tract
fasciotomy, anterior compartment
fashion
   antegrade
   retrograde
FAST (flow-assisted, short-term)
FAST balloon catheter
Fast-Pass lead pacemaker
fat
   animal (in diet)
   epicardial
   monounsaturated
   polyunsaturated
   preperitoneal
   properitoneal
   saturated
   unsaturated
fatigability, easy
Favaloro sternal retractor
Favaloro-Morse rib spreader
fear of impending death feeling from angina
febrile agglutinins
feeling of impending doom prior to MI (myocardial infarction)
feet, cold
Feigenbaum echocardiogram
felt bolster, Teflon
felt strip
fem-pop (femoral-popliteal) bypass
femoral approach for cardiac catheterization
femoral-femoral crossover
femoral vein
femoral pulse
femoral-peroneal in situ vein bypass graft
femoral-popliteal Gore-Tex graft
femoroaxillary bypass
femorodistal bypass
femorofemoral bypass

femoropopliteal bypass surgery
femorotibial bypass
fenestration, cusp
Ferguson forceps
ferrule (on pacemaker wires)
FFA (free fatty acid) scintigraphy,
  labeled
FHC (familial hypertrophic cardiomyopathy)
fiber, fibers
  accelerating
  atrio-Hisian
  Brechenmacher
  bystander
  cardiac accelerator
  cardiac depressor
  cardiac muscle
  cardiac pressor
  depressor
  dietary
  fasciculoventricular bypass
  fasciculoventricular Mahaim
  impulse conducting
  James
  Kent
  Mahaim
  muscle
  nodoventricular bypass
  Purkinje
fiber-shortening velocity (V$_{CF}$)
fibrillation
  atrial (AF)
  auricular
  ventricular (VF)
fibrillation-flutter
fibrillation rhythm
fibrillator, electric
fibrin glue sealant
fibrin stabilizing blood coagulation
  factor
fibrinogen, technetium^{99m} labeled
fibrinogen-fibrin conversion
  syndrome
fibrinolysis of thrombi
fibrinous exudate

fibroelastoma of heart valve
fibroelastosis, endocardial
fibroma of heart
fibrosarcoma of heart
fibrosa, intervalvular
fibrosis
  African endomyocardial
  bundle branch
  Davies endomyocardial
  diffuse interstitial pulmonary
    (DIPF)
  endocardial
  endomyocardial (EMF)
  idiopathic pulmonary (IPF)
  myocardial
  nodal
  perielectrode
  pulmonary
  rheumatic
fibrotic mitral valve
Fick cardiac output and index
Fick cardiac output method
  assumed
  direct
Fick principle
field
  bloodless
  surgical
FILE (Family Index of Life Events)
filiform pulse
filling
  capillary
  rapid (RF)
  retrograde
  ventricular
filling pressure
filter
  caval
  Greenfield
  Kim-Ray Greenfield caval
  Mobin-Uddin umbrella
  umbrella
Finesse large-lumen guiding catheter
finger fracture dissection
finned pacemaker lead

Finochietto forceps
Finochietto retractor
Finochietto rib spreader
Finochietto thoracic scissors
FiO$_2$ (forced inspiratory oxygen)
first-pass study
Fischer sign
fishhook lead
fistula
   aortic sinus
   aorto-left ventricular
   aorto-right ventricular
   arteriovenous (AVF)
   AV (arteriovenous)
   Brescio-Cimino AV
   carotid-cavernous
   coronary arteriovenous
   coronary artery to right
      ventricular
   coronary artery-pulmonary
      artery
   coronary-cameral
   coronary-pulmonary
   intrapulmonary arteriovenous
   pulmonary arteriovenous
Fitzgerald aortic aneurysm forceps
Flack node
FL4 guide
flail mitral leaflet
flail mitral valve
flank incision
flap
   pericardial
   scimitar-shaped
   Waldenhausen subclavian
FLASH (fast low-angle shot) cardiac MRI
flat-hand test
flat lined (verb)
flat neck veins
flat P wave
flattening of ST segment
Flex guide wire
Flexguide intubation guide
flexible J guide wire
flexible steerable wire
Flexon steel suture
flip, LDH$_1$
flip-flop of heart
flipped T wave
floppy mitral valve syndrome
Flo-Rester vessel occluder
flotation catheter
flow
   antegrade diastolic
   aortic (AF)
   blood
   cerebral blood (CBF)
   chronic reserve
   collateral
   coronary reserve (CRF)
   effective pulmonary blood
      (EPBF)
   effective pulmonic
   forward
   Ganz method for coronary sinus
   great cardiac vein (GCVF)
   high velocity
   laminar
   left-to-right
   mitral valve
   myocardial blood (MBF)
   pulmonary blood (PBF)
   pulmonic output
   pulmonic versus systemic
   redistribution of pulmonary
      vascular
   regional myocardial blood
   regurgitant systolic
   restoration of
   retrograde systolic
   reversed vertebral blood (RVBF)
   sluggish
   systemic blood (SBF)
   systemic output
   total cerebral blood (TCBF)
   transmitral
   tricuspid valve
   turbulent blood
flow-directed

flow mapping technique
flow velocity profile
flowmeter
   Narcomatic
   Parks 800 bidirectional Doppler
   Statham electromagnetic
fluid challenge
fluid, pericardial
fluorescein angiography
fluorine-18 deoxyglucose
fluoroscopic control, advanced under
fluoroscopic guidance
Fluosol (artificial blood)
Fluosol-DA 20% (oxygen transport fluid)
flush
   heparinized saline
   malar
flush aortogram
flushing of catheter
flutter
   atrial (AFl)
   auricular
   coarse atrial
   impure
   pure
   ventricular
fluttering of valvular leaflet
flutter-fibrillation
focal eccentric stenosis
focal wall motion abnormality
Foerster forceps
Fogarty arterial embolectomy catheter
Fogarty balloon catheter
Fogarty forceps
Fogarty Hydrogrip clamp
Fogarty occlusion catheter
Fogarty venous thrombectomy catheter
Fogarty-Chin clamp; clip
Fogarty-Chin extrusion balloon catheter
fold of Rindfleisch

Fontan modification of Norwood procedure
Fontan operation for tricuspid atresia and pulmonary stenosis
Fontan-Kreutzer operation
Fontan-Kreutzer repair, modified
foot cradle
foramen of Morgagni
foramen ovale, patent
foramen secundum
force, lateral anterior
forceps
   Adson
   alligator
   Allis
   artery
   Bailey aortic valve cutting
   Bengolea artery
   Bloodwell
   Boettcher artery
   bronchus
   Brown Adson
   Brunschwig artery
   bulldog
   Carmalt artery
   Cooley vascular
   Cooley-Baumgarten aortic
   Crile
   Cushing
   Dale
   Davis
   DeBakey arterial
   DeBakey Autaugrip
   DeBakey dissecting
   DeBakey tissue
   DeBakey vascular
   DeBakey-Diethrich vascular
   DeBakey-Semb
   Duval lung
   Duval-Crile lung
   Effler-Groves
   Ferguson
   Finochietto
   Fitzgerald aortic aneurysm
   Foerster

forceps *(cont.)*
   Fogarty
   Foss
   Gemini thoracic
   Gerald
   Gerbode
   grasping
   Halstead
   Harrington thoracic
   Harrington-Mixter thoracic
   Hayes Martin
   Heiss artery
   hemoclip-applying
   hemostatic
   Hendrin
   Hopkins aortic
   Johns Hopkins
   Johnson thoracic
   Jones IMA
   Julian thoracic
   Karp aortic punch
   Lahey thoracic
   Lees artery
   Lejeune thoracic
   Lillehei valve
   Mayo Pean
   Mixter
   mosquito
   NIH mitral valve
   Ochsner
   O'Shaughnessy artery
   Overholt thoracic
   Phaneuf artery
   Potts bronchus
   Potts bulldog
   Potts thumb
   Potts vascular
   Potts-Smith tissue
   Price-Thomas bronchial
   Randall stone
   Rochester-Mixter artery
   Ruel
   Rumel thoracic
   Russian tissue
   Samuels

forceps *(cont.)*
   Sarot artery
   Selman vessel
   Semb
   Singley
   Snowden-Pencer
   sponge
   straight-end cup
   Thomas Allis
   thumb
   tissue
   tonsillar
   torsion
   Tuttle thoracic
   up-biting cup
   Westphal
   Yasargil artery
forme fruste
formula (see also *method*)
   Ganz coronary sinus flow
   Gorlin valve area
   Hakki
Forrester syndrome
Forrester Therapeutic Class
forward flow of velocity
forward triangle method
Foss forceps
fossa
   antecubital
   cardiac
fossa ovalis cordis
four-chamber apical view
four-chamber plane on echocardiography
Fourier analysis of electrocardiogram
Fowler position
Fox green dye
fraction (see also *ejection fraction*)
   beta lipoprotein
   MB
   MM
   regurgitant
fractional area
fractional shortening, percentage of

fracture, annular
Framingham Data; Study
frank blood
Frank EKG lead system placement
Frank-Starling principle
Frank XYZ orthogonal lead system
Frantzel murmur
Frazier suction tip; tube
Fredrickson classification of hyperlipoproteinemia
free end of electrode
freeing up of adhesions
Freer elevator
French 5 angiographic catheter
French MBIH catheter
French scale for caliber of catheter
friable wall
friction rub
Friedländer (Friedlaender) disease
Friedreich sign
FRP (functional refractory period)
   atrial
   ventricular
frontal plane on EKG
frontotemporal muscle

FSV (forward stroke volume)
fulcrum, left ventricular
fulguration, endocavitary
fulguration during electrophysiologic study
fulminant
function
   exercise LV
   global left ventricular
   left ventricular (LV)
   left ventricular systolic/diastolic
   left ventricular systolic pump
   regional left ventricular
   reserve cardiac
   rest LV
   rest RV
   right ventricular (RV)
   right ventricular systolic/diastolic
   ventricular contractility (VCF)
functional aerobic impairment (FAI)
functional classification of CHF
functional refractory period (FRP)
funduscopy, funduscopic
fusion QRS complex

G

G suit (for syncope)
Gaertner phenomenon
Gairdner disease
Galaxy pacemaker
Gallavardin murmur; phenomenon
gallium-67
gallop
   atrial
   early diastolic
   low-frequency
   presystolic atrial
   S_3 (third heart sound)

gallop *(cont.)*
   S_4 (fourth heart sound)
   summation
   systolic
   ventricular
   ventricular diastolic
gallop, murmur, or rub (GMR)
ganglionectomy, left stellate
Ganz formula for coronary sinus flow
Ganz-Edwards coronary infusion catheter

Garcia aorta clamp
Garrett dilator
Garrett retractor
Garrett vascular dilator
gas, arterial blood (ABG) (see *blood gas*)
gastrocardiac syndrome
gated blood (pool) cardiac wall motion study
gated blood pool ventriculogram
gated cardiac blood pool imaging
gated equilibrium blood pool scanning
gating of heartbeats
gauze, Surgicel
GCVF (great cardiac vein flow)
gel
    EKG
    electrode
    Lectron II electrode
gelatin compression boot
gelatinous debris
Gelfilm
Gelfoam
Gelfoam soaked in thrombin
Gelpi retractor
Gemini 415 DDD pacemaker
Gemini thoracic forceps
General Electric Pass-C echocardiograph machine
General Electric pacemaker
generator (see also *pacemaker*)
    asynchronous
    Aurora pulse
    bipolar
    Chardack-Greatbatch implantable cardiac pulse
    Cosmos pulse
    Cyberlith multi-programmable pulse
    fixed rate
    implantable pulse
    intrapleural pulse
    lithium-powered pulse
    Medtronics demand pulse

generator *(cont.)*
    multiprogrammable pulse
    physiologic
    Programalith III pulse
    pulse
    Spectrax SXT pulse
    subpectoral pulse
    Telectronics PASAR antitachycardia pulse
    ventricular demand
    ventricular inhibited pulse
    Versatrax pulse
Genisis pacemaker
Gensini catheter
Gensini scoring of coronary artery disease
Gentle-Flo suction catheter
Gentran 40; 75
Gerald forceps
Gerbode dilator
Gerbode forceps
Gerbode mitral valvulotome
Gerbode patent ductus clamp
Gerbode valve dilator
giant cell aortitis; arteritis
giant cell myocarditis
Gianturco wool-tufted wire coil; stent
Gibbon and Landis test
Gibson murmur
Giertz rongeur
Gigli saw
Gill-Jonas modification of Norwood procedure
Glasgow sign
Glenn anastomosis
Glenn shunt
Glidewire
global cardiac disease
global ejection fraction
global left ventricular function
global ventricular dysfunction
globoid heart
globulin, rabbit antithymocyte (RATG)

Glover coarctation clamp
Glover patent ductus clamp
Glover vascular clamp
Gluck rib shears
glutaraldehyde-tanned bovine collagen tubes for grafts
glutaraldehyde-tanned porcine heart valve
GMR (gallop, murmur, or rub)
Goethlin test
gold-195m radionuclide
Goldblatt hypertension
Goldblatt phenomenon
Goldenhar syndrome
Goodale-Lubin catheter
Goosen vascular punch
gooseneck deformity of outflow tract (on x-ray)
Gore-Tex bifurcated vascular graft
Gore-Tex cardiovascular patch
Gore-Tex catheter
Gore-Tex graft; limb; shunt
Gore-Tex soft tissue patch
Gore-Tex surgical membrane
Gore-Tex vascular graft
Gorlin catheter
Gorlin formula for aortic valve area
Gorlin hydraulic formula for mitral valve area
Gorlin method for cardiac output
Gorlin pacing catheter
Gott shunt/butterfly heart valve
Gould PentaCath 5-lumen thermodilution catheter
Gould Statham pressure transducer
grade 2-3/6 (or II-III/VI) holosystolic murmur
gradient
   aortic outflow
   aortic valve (AVG)
   aortic valve peak instantaneous
   brain-core
   coronary perfusion
   diastolic
   elevated

gradient *(cont.)*
   end-diastolic aortic-left ventricular pressure
   holosystolic
   instantaneous
   left ventricular outflow pressure
   maximal estimated
   mean mitral valve
   mean systolic
   mitral valve
   outflow tract
   peak diastolic
   peak instantaneous
   peak pressure
   peak right ventricular-right atrial systolic
   peak systolic (PSG)
   peak-to-peak pressure
   pressure
   pulmonary artery diastolic and wedge pressure (PADP-PAWP)
   pulmonary artery to right ventricle diastolic
   pulmonary outflow
   pulmonic valve
   residual
   right ventricular to main pulmonary artery pressure
   stenotic
   subvalvular
   systolic
   transaortic systolic
   translesional
   transmitral diastolic
   transpulmonic
   transstenotic pressure
   transtricuspid valve diastolic
   transvalvular pressure
   tricuspid valve
   ventricular
gradient across valve
graft
   albumin coated vascular
   aorta to left anterior descending saphenous vein bypass

graft *(cont.)*
 aortocoronary bypass
 aortocoronary snake
 aortofemoral bypass (AFBG)
 autologous vein
 bifurcated vascular
 bifurcation
 Biograft
 bovine allograft
 bovine heterograft
 bypass
 composite valve
 coronary artery bypass (CABG)
 cryopreserved human aortic allograft
 Dacron knitted
 Dacron onlay patch
 Dacron patch
 Dacron preclotted
 Dacron tightly woven
 Dacron tube
 Dacron tubular
 Dacron velour
 deaired
 double velour knitted
 endothelialization of vascular
 extracardiac
 extrathoracic carotid subclavian bypass
 femoral-peroneal in situ vein bypass
 femoro-distal vein
 glutaraldehyde-tanned bovine carotid artery
 glutaraldehyde-tanned bovine collagen tubes for vascular
 glutaraldehyde-tanned porcine heart valve
 Gore-Tex bifurcated vascular
 Gore-Tex jump
 Hancock pericardial valve
 heterograft
 homograft
 human umbilical vein (HUV) bypass

graft *(cont.)*
 HUV (human umbilical vein) bypass
 IMA (internal mammary artery)
 internal mammary artery (IMA)
 internal thoracic artery (ITA)
 Ionescu-Shiley pericardial valve
 ITA (internal thoracic artery)
 jump
 kinking of
 knitted
 knitted Dacron arterial
 LIMA (left internal mammary artery)
 Meadox Microvel
 modified human umbilical vein (HUV)
 nonvalved
 patch
 patent
 Plasma TFE vascular
 porcine xenograft
 preclotted
 prosthetic patch
 PTFE (polytetrafluoroethylene)
 saphenous vein (SVG) bypass
 Sauvage
 sequential
 snake
 St. Jude composite valve
 straight
 straight tubular
 synthetic
 Teflon
 tube
 umbilical vein
 unilateral aortofemoral
 valved
 vein patch
 ventriculoarterial
 woven Dacron
 Y-shaped
graft dependent
graft insertion site
graft occlusion

graft occlusive disease
graft-patch
graft patency
graft-seeking catheter
graft trimmed on the bias
graftable
grafting (see *graft*)
Graham Steell heart murmur
Gram stain
Grancher sign
Grant aneurysm clamp
GRASS (gradient recalled acquisition in steady state)
Graupner method
great vessel, orientation of
greater saphenous vein
Greene sign
Greenfield filter
Gregg-type cannula
Gregory baby profunda clamp
Gregory carotid bulldog clamp
Gregory external clamp
Gregory forceps
Gregory stay suture
Grocco sign
groin area
Grollman catheter
groove
    anterior interventricular
    atrioventricular (AV)
    deltopectoral
    interatrial
    interventricular
    posterior interventricular
    Waterston
Groshong double-lumen catheter
Gross coarctation occlusion clamp
Grossman scale for regurgitation
Grossman sign
Grover clamp
growth retardation
Gruentzig balloon catheter angioplasty
Gruentzig Dilaca catheter
Gruentzig technique for PTCA

grumose, grumous material
Guangzhou GD-1 prosthetic valve
Guardian pacemaker
guide
    ACS LIMA
    Amplatz
    Arani
    FL4
    Flexguide intubation
    Muller catheter
    Pilotip catheter
    steerable wire
guide wire (guidewire)
    ACS (Advanced Catheter Systems)
    Amplatz Super Stiff
    angiographic
    Bentson floppy-tip
    Flex
    flexible
    flexible J
    floppy
    floppy-tipped
    high torque
    Hi-Per Flex
    Hi-Torque Flex-T
    Hi-Torque Floppy (HTF)
    Hi-Torque Intermediate
    Hi-Torque Standard
    J
    J tip
    J-tipped exchange
    Linx exchange
    PDT
    Redifocus
    Rosen
    Schwarten LP
    Sof-T
    soft-tipped
    Sones
    SOS
    steerable
    straight
    TAD
    Teflon-coated

guide wire *(cont.)*
   transluminal coronary angio-
     plasty
   USCI
   VeriFlex
   Wholey Hi-Torque Floppy
   Wholey Hi-Torque Modified J

guide wire *(cont.)*
   Wholey Hi-Torque Standard
guiding catheter
guillotine, rib
Gunn crossing sign
Gutgeman clamp

H

H spike
H' (H prime) spike
H&H (hemoglobin and hematocrit)
H'P interval
h peak of jugular venous pulse
h plateau of jugular venous pulse
h wave of jugular venous pulse
Haemonetics Cell Saver System
Hagar probe
Hageman blood coagulation factor
Haight rib spreader
Haight-Finochietto rib retractor
Haimovici arteriotomy scissors
hair growth
   decreased lower leg
     distribution of
hair loss
Hakki formula
Hall prosthetic heart valve
Hall sign
Hall sternal saw
Hall-Kaster mitral valve prosthesis
Hall-Kaster tilting-disk valve
   prosthesis
Halstead forceps
Hamman crunch; murmur; sign
Hamman-Rich syndrome
hammocking of leaflet
hammocking of mitral valve
Hanafee catheter

Hancock aortic bioprosthesis
Hancock aortic punch
Hancock bioprosthetic valve
Hancock conduit
Hancock mitral valve prosthesis
Hancock pericardial prosthetic valve
Hancock porcine heterograft valve
Hancock valved conduit
hand-agitated contrast medium
hand-agitated solution with micro-
   bubbles
hand injection
handgrip exercise test
hand-made injection
hang-out of dicrotic notch in pul-
   monary arterial pressure
Hank balanced salt solution
hardening of arteries
Harken auricle clamp
Harken prosthetic valve
Harken rib spreader
Harrington retractor
Harrington thoracic forceps
Harrington-Mayo thoracic scissors
Harrington-Mixter thoracic forceps
Hartzler angioplasty balloon
Hartzler LPS dilatation catheter
Hartzler Micro II catheter
Hartzler Micro XT dilatation
   catheter

Hartzler rib retractor
harvest(ing) vein, tissue, or organ from donor for transplantation
Hatle method to calculate mitral valve area
Hayes Martin forceps
Haynes 25 material for prosthetic valve construction
HBE (His bundle electrogram)
HBP (high blood pressure)
HCM (hypertrophic cardiomyopathy)
HCT (hematocrit)
HCVD (hypertensive cardiovascular disease)
H-DCSA (His bundle-distal coronary sinus atrial) depolarization
HDL (high-density lipoprotein)
headhunter catheter
heart
  abdominal
  Akutsu total artificial
  armored
  artificial
  athlete's
  athletic
  balloon-shaped
  beer
  beriberi
  boat-shaped
  bony
  booster
  boot-shaped (on x-ray)
  bovine
  chaotic
  cervical
  donor
  dynamite
  encased
  enlarged
  extracorporeal
  fatty
  fibroid
  flask-shaped
  frosted (frosting; icing)

heart *(cont.)*
  globoid
  hairy
  hanging (suspended)
  holiday
  horizontal
  hyperthyroid
  hypoplastic
  icing (frosting)
  intracorporeal
  irritable
  Jarvik 7 or 8 artificial
  Jarvik 7-70 artificial
  left (atrium and ventricle)
  Liotta total artificial
  luxus
  mechanical
  movable
  myxedema
  one-ventricle
  orthotopic biventricular artificial
  orthotopic univentricular artificial
  ox
  paracorporeal
  parchment
  pear-shaped
  pectoral
  pendulous
  Penn State total artificial
  Phoenix total artificial
  pulmonary
  Quain fatty
  recipient
  right (atrium and ventricle)
  round
  sabot
  semihorizontal
  semivertical
  skin (peripheral blood vessels)
  snowman (on x-ray)
  soldier's
  stiff
  stone
  suspended

heart (cont.)
   systemic
   tabby cat
   teardrop
   three-chambered
   thrush breast
   tiger
   tiger lily
   tobacco
   total artificial (TAH)
   Traube
   triatrial
   trilocular
   univentricular
   Utah artificial
   Utah TAH
   venous
   vertical
   wandering
   wooden shoe
Heart Aid 80 defibrillator
heart and great vessels
heart attack
heartbeat (see also *beat*)
   coupling
   dropped
   fluttering
   irregular
   irregularly irregular
   pounding
   racing
   regular
   skipping
heart block (see *block*)
heartburn (pyrosis; water brash)
heart-lung bloc
heart-lung machine
heart-lung transplant
heart murmur (see *murmur*)
heart overload
heart rate (see *rate*)
heart rate response
heart sound (see *sound*)
heart tones (sounds)
heart valve (see *valve; prosthesis*)

heave
   parasternal
   substernal
heave and lift
heaviness, chest
heaving of chest wall
Heberden angina
Heberden disease
Hegar dilator
Hegglin syndrome
Heifitz clip
Heim-Kreysig sign
Heinz body
Heiss artery forceps
hemangioma-thrombocytopenia
   syndrome
hemangiopericytoma
Hemaquet catheter introducer
Hemaquet sheath introducer
hematemesis
hematocrit (HCT)
hematoma, mural
hematopoiesis
Hemex prosthetic valve
hemiblock
   left anterior-posterior
   left anterior-superior (LASH)
   left posterior (LPH)
hemithymectomy
hemochromatosis
hemoclip, Samuels
HemoCue photometer for hemoglobin determination
hemodilution, intentional transoperative
hemodynamic assessment
hemodynamic data
hemodynamic effect
hemodynamic instability
hemodynamic monitoring, continuous
hemodynamic significance
hemodynamically significant lesions
hemodynamics, cardiovascular
hemoglobin (Hgb)

hemoglobin and hematocrit (H&H)
hemoglobin, stroma free (SFHb)
Hemopad
hemopericardium
hemophilia A
hemophilia B
hemophilia, vascular
hemopleuropneumonia syndrome
hemoptysis
hemorrhage
   arterial
   capillary
   exsanguinating
   external
   internal
   intraplaque (IPH)
   splinter
   venous
hemosiderosis
hemostasis, hemostatic
hemostat (see also *forceps*)
   Crile
   Kelly
   Mayo
   mosquito
   Woodward
hematoma, retroperitoneal
Hendrin ductus clamp; forceps
Henle-Coenen test
Henley dilator; vascular clamp
heparin, neutralize the effects of
heparin lock introducer
heparin lock for administering medication
heparin reversed with protamine
heparinization, systemic
heparinized blood
heparinized saline flush
hepatic vein pulsation
hepatojugular reflux
Hercules power injector
hereditary pseudohemophilia
Hering, nerve of
hermetically sealed standby pacemaker

hernia, intrapericardial diaphragmatic
Hershey left ventricular assist device
Hespan (hetastarch) plasma volume expander
Hess capillary test
hetastarch (Hespan)
heterogeneity, temporal
heterograft (see also *graft*)
   bovine
   porcine
heterotaxy, visceral
Hetzel forward triangle method for cardiac output
Heubner disease
Hewlett-Packard color flow imager
Hewlett-Packard defibrillator
Hewlett-Packard transducer
Hewlett-Packard ultrasound
Hexabrix contrast medium
HFD40 (duration of terminal QRS high frequency signal)
HFQRSD (duration of high frequency QRS)
HFRMS (voltage of terminal QRS high frequency signal)
Hgb (hemoglobin)
H&H (hemoglobin and hematocrit)
HH' interval
HHD (hypertensive heart disease)
Hickman indwelling right atrial catheter
Hidalgo catheter
Hiebert vascular dilator
high blood pressure (HBP)
high-density lipoprotein (HDL)
high-grade lesion
high-grade stenosis
high left main diagonal artery
high right atrium
high torque (see *Hi-Torque*)
hilar haze
Hill sign
Hi-Lo Jet tracheal tube
Himmelstein sternal retractor

Himmelstein valvulotome
Hines and Brown test
hinge, annulocuspid
Hi-Per Flex guide wire
His bundle electrogram (HBE)
His-Purkinje system (HPS)
histogram, plasma
Histoplasma myocarditis
Hi-Torque Flex-T guide wire
Hi-Torque Floppy (HTF) guide wire
Hi-Torque Intermediate guide wire
Hi-Torque Standard guide wire
HLHS (hypoplastic left heart syndrome)
H-MCSA (His bundle-middle coronary sinus atrial) depolarization
HMG CoA reductase inhibitor
HOC or HOCM (hypertrophic obstructive cardiomyopathy)
hockey-stick deformity of cusp (on echocardiogram)
hockey-stick deformity of tricuspid valve
Hodgkin-Key murmur
Hodgson disease
Hoen nerve hook
Hohn vessel dilator
holder
  needle
  prosthetic valve
  valve
  wire needle
holiday heart syndrome
Holinger dissector
holosystolic murmur
Holt-Oram syndrome
Holter monitor
Holter monitoring, continuous
Holter shunt; tubing; valve
Homans sign
Hombach lead placement system
homocystinuria, congenital
homogeneous thallium distribution
homograft, cryopreserved
homograft conduit

homonymous
honk, precordial
hooding, interchordal
hook
  Adson
  Hoen nerve
  Krayenbuehl vessel
  nerve
  Selverstone cardiotomy valve
Hope sign
Hopkins aortic clamp; forceps
horizontal mattress suture
horizontal ST segment depression
horseshoe configuration on thallium imaging
Horton disease
Howell coronary scissors
Howell test
H-PCSA (His bundle-proximal coronary sinus atrial depolarization)
HPS (His-Purkinje system)
HQ interval
H-QRS interval
HR (heart rate) (beats/min)
HRA (high right atrium)
HTN (hypertension)
Huchard disease; sign
Hufnagel aortic clamp
Hufnagel prosthetic valve
hum, venous
Humphries aortic clamp
Hunter canal
Hunter operation for correction of aneurysm
Hunter-Sessions balloon
Hunter-Sessions inferior vena cava balloon occluder
Hurwitz thoracic trocar
HUV (human umbilical vein) bypass graft
H-V (His-ventricular) interval
Hx (history)
HydraCross TLC PTCA catheter
hydrate(d), hydration

Hypaque Meglumine
Hypaque Sodium contrast medium
Hypaque-76 contrast medium
Hypaque-M contrast medium
hyperabduction maneuver
hyperalphalipoproteinemia
hypercapnia
hypercholesterolemia
   familial
   polygenic
hyperkinesia, compensatory
hyperkinetic
hyperlipidemia
   combined
   familial
   familial combined
   mixed
   multiple lipoprotein-type
   remnant
hyperlipoproteinemia
hyperosmotic solution
hyperplasia, intimal
hypersensitivity, carotid sinus (CHS)
hypertension (HTN)
   accelerated
   adrenal
   arterial (AHT)
   borderline
   continued arterial
   disproportionate femoral systolic
   essential
   glucocorticoid-induced
   Goldblatt
   hypoxic pulmonary
   idiopathic
   labile
   long-standing
   low-renin
   malignant
   mineralocorticoid-induced
   oral contraceptive-induced
   pale
   portal
   pregnancy-induced
   primary

hypertension *(cont.)*
   primary pulmonary (PPH)
   pulmonary
   pulmonary arterial
   pulmonary artery
   pulmonary thromboembolic
   pulmonary venous
   pulmonary (PHTN)
   red
   renal
   renovascular
   secondary
   symptomatic
   systemic venous
   systolic
   thromboembolic pulmonary
   vascular
   white-coat (fear of doctors)
hypertensive crisis
hypertensive emergency
hypertensive encephalopathy
hypertriglyceridemia
   carbohydrate-induced
   endogenous
   familial
hypertrophic obstructive cardiomyopathy (HOC or HOCM)
hypertrophy
   asymmetric septal (ASH)
   biatrial
   biventricular
   compensatory
   concentric
   concentric left ventricular
   eccentric left ventricular
   four-chamber
   hypertrophic
   left atrial
   left ventricular (LVH)
   myocardial cellular
   panchamber
   right atrial
   right ventricular (RVH)
   type A right ventricular
   type B right ventricular

hypertrophy (cont.)
   type C right ventricular
   unilateral
   ventricular
   Wigle scale for ventricular
hypocontractility
hypogastric artery
hypogastric system
hypokalemia-induced arrhythmia
hypokinesia
   diffuse
   regional
hypokinesis
   apical
   diffuse
   diffuse ventricular
   hypokinetic
   inferior wall
hypokinetic left ventricle
hyponatremia
hypoperfusion
   apical
   peripheral
   septal
hypoplastic left-sided heart syndrome (HLHS)
hypotension
   chronic orthostatic
   exercise-induced
   exertional
   idiopathic orthostatic
   orthostatic
   postural
   stress-induced
   vascular
hypothermia
   deep
   endogenous
   local
   myocardial
   profound
   surface
   systemic and topical
   topical
   total body
hypothermia blanket
hypovolemia, hypovolemic
hypoxemia
hypoxia, hypoxic
hysteresis
   AV delay (AVDH)
   rate

I

IAB (intra-aortic balloon) catheter
IABP (intra-aortic balloon pump)
IAS (interatrial septum)
IAVB (incomplete atrioventricular block)
IAVD (incomplete atrioventricular dissociation)
ICA (internal carotid artery)
ice slush
ice, topical
ice-pick view on M-mode echocardiogram
ICHD (Inter-Society Commission for Heart Disease)
ICHD pacemaker code
ICRBBB (incomplete right bundle branch block)
ICU (intensive care unit)
IDC (idiopathic dilated cardiomyopathy)
idiopathic bradycardia
idiopathic hypertrophic subaortic stenosis (IHSS)
idiopathic orthostatic hypotension
IDL (intermediate density lipoprotein)
IDSA (intraoperative digital subtraction angiography)

IHSS (idiopathic hypertrophic subaortic stenosis)
IJV (internal jugular vein)
ILBBB (incomplete left bundle
   branch block)
iliac atherosclerotic occlusive disease
iliac fossa
iliac vessel
iliopopliteal bypass
IMA (internal mammary artery)
   graft; pedicle
image, imaging (see also *scan*)
   antifibrin antibody
   cardiac blood pool
   color flow
   delayed
   Doppler color flow
   ED (end-diastolic)
   four-hour delayed thallium
   gated cardiac blood pool
   indium-111 antimyosin imaging
   infarct avid
   initial
   magnetic resonance (MRI)
   myocardial perfusion
   myocardial Tl
   multiple gated equilibrium car-
      diac blood pool
   postexercise
   radioisotope
   redistribution myocardial
   redistribution thallium-201
   regional ejection fraction (REFI)
   rest myocardial perfusion
   rest thallium-201 myocardial
   rubidium-82
   stress thallium-201 myocardial
   Tc myocardial
   technetium[99m] pyrophosphate
      myocardial
   thallium-201 myocardial
   thallium myocardial perfusion
   Tl myocardial
   transesophageal Doppler color
      flow
   imager, Hewlett-Packard color flow
IMI (inferior myocardial infarction)
impairment of contractility
impedance plethysmography (IPG)
impedance
   pacemaker lead
   pulmonary arterial input
implantable system
implantation
   intrapleural pulse generator
   permanent pacemaker
   subpectoral pulse generator
impulse
   apical
   atrial filling
   cardiac
   cardiac apex
   episternal
   juxtapical
   left parasternal
   paradoxic apical
   point of maximal (PMI)
   right parasternal
IMV (intermittent mandatory ventilation)
in extremis
in situ bypass
in situ grafting
in toto
in vivo balloon pressure
incentive spirometry
incision
   flank
   longitudinal
   median sternotomy
   pleuropericardial
   stab
   stepladder
   submammary
   thoracicoabdominal
   thoracoabdominal
   transverse
   xiphoid to os pubis
incisura apicis cordis
incisura of carotid arterial pulse

inclination of the treadmill
inclusion technique of Bentall
incompetence
  aortic valve
  valve
incomplete atrioventricular block (IAVB); dissociation (IAVD)
increase in heart rate
Ind (indeterminate)
Indeflator, ACS
indeterminate age
index, indices
  angiographic muscle mass
  ankle-arm
  ankle-brachial (ABI)
  body mass
  cardiac (CI)
  cardiothoracic
  contractile work
  contractility
  coronary stenosis (CSI)
  coronary vascular resistance (CVRI)
  diastolic left ventricular
  diastolic pressure-time (DPTI)
  effective pulmonic
  end-diastolic volume (EDVI)
  end-systolic stress wall (ESWI)
  end-systolic volume (ESVI)
  Fick cardiac
  FILE (Family Index of Life Events)
  Fourmentin thoracic
  hemodynamic
  left ventricular end-diastolic volume (LVEDI)
  left ventricular end-systolic volume (LVESVI)
  left ventricular fractional shortening
  left ventricular mass (LVMI)
  left ventricular stroke volume
  left ventricular stroke work
  mean ankle-brachial systolic pressure

index *(cont.)*
  mean wall motion score
  mitral flow velocity
  myocardial infarction recovery (MIRI)
  myocardial jeopardy
  myocardial O_2 demand
  O_2 consumption
  penile-brachial pressure (PBPI)
  postexercise (PEI)
  pulmonary arterial resistance
  pulmonary blood volume (PBVI)
  pulmonic output
  QOL (quality of life)
  regurgitant
  resting ankle-arm pressure (RAAPI)
  right and left ankle
  stroke (SI)
  stroke volume (SVI)
  stroke work (SWI)
  systemic arteriolar resistance
  systemic output
  tension-time (TTI)
  thoracic
  venous distensibility (VDI)
  wall motion score
  Wood units
indicator dilution curve; method; technique
indicator fractionation principle
indices (see *index*)
indium-111 antimyosin antibody
indium-111 antimyosin imaging
indium-111 radioisotope
indium-111 scintigraphy
indium-113m
indocyanine dilution curve
indocyanine green dye
inducibility, VT (ventricular tachycardia)
inducibility basal state
inducible sustained orthodromic supraventricular tachycardia
induction of anesthesia, crash

Inf (infarction)
infarct expansion
infarct size limitation
infarctectomy
infarction
    acute myocardial (AMI)
    age indeterminate
    anterior myocardial (AMI)
    anteroinferior myocardial
    anterolateral myocardial
    anteroseptal myocardial
    arrhythmic myocardial
    atherothrombotic
    atrial
    cardiac
    diaphragmatic myocardial (DMI)
    evolving myocardial
    hyperacute myocardial
    impending myocardial
    inferior myocardial (IMI)
    inferolateral myocardial
    inferoposterolateral myocardial
    lateral myocardial
    myocardial (MI)
    nonarrhythmic myocardial
    nonfatal myocardial
    nontransmural myocardial
    non-Q wave myocardial
    old myocardial
    posterior myocardial
    posteroinferior myocardial
    postmyocardial
    postmyocardiotomy
    Q wave myocardial
    recent myocardial
    septal myocardial
    silent myocardial
    subacute myocardial
    subendocardial (SEI)
    subendocardial myocardial
    transmural myocardial
infarctoid cardiopathy
infective endocarditis
inferior vena cava (IVC)
inferior wall hypokinesis
inferior wall MI (myocardial infarction)
inferobasal
inferolateral
inferoposterior
inferoposterolateral
inflammation, fibrinous
inflow tract of left ventricle
infra-apical
infra-auricular
infraclavicular
inframyocardial
infundibular resection
infundibulectomy
infundibuloventricular crest
infundibulum
infusion, volume
inguinal region
injection
    bolus
    double
    hand
    intra-arterial
    intramuscular (I.M.)
    intravascular
    intravenous (I.V.)
    manual
    opacifying
    power
    sclerosing
    selective
    serial
    straight AP pelvic
injection port
injector
    Hercules power
    Medrad power angiographic
innominate artery stenosis
Innovator Holter system
inotropic activity of drug
inotropic agent; effect; therapy
Inoue balloon catheter
instantaneous gradient
instrumentation
instrumented

insufficiency
   acute coronary
   aortic (AI)
   aortic valve
   cardiac
   congenital pulmonary valve
   coronary
   mitral (MI)
   myocardial (MI)
   nonrheumatic aortic
   pulmonary (PI)
   renal
   Sternberg myocardial
   tricuspid (TI)
   valvular
   venous
   vertebrobasilar arterial
Intact xenograft prosthetic valve
Intec implantable defibrillator
integral
   aortic flow velocity
   pulmonary flow velocity
intensity of heart sounds
intensive care unit (ICU)
intentional transoperative hemodilution
interatrial baffle leak
interatrial septal defect
interchordal hooding
intercostal artery
intermediate artery
Intermedics Quantum pacemaker
intermittent claudication
intermittent junctional bradycardia
internal jugular approach for cardiac catheterization
internodal pathway; tract
interpolated premature complex
Intertach 262-12 pacemaker
interval
   A_1A_2
   A_2 incisural
   A_2 to opening snap
   A_2/MVO (aortic valve closure/mitral valve opening)

interval (cont.)
   AA
   AC
   Ae-H
   AH
   atrial escape (AEI)
   atrioventricular
   AV delay (AVDI)
   cardioarterial
   coupling
   fixed coupling
   flutter R
   H_1H_2
   HH'
   H'P
   HQ
   H-QRS
   HV
   interectopic
   isoelectric
   P_2T_0
   PA
   pacemaker escape
   PH
   PP
   PR
   prolongation of QRS
   QH
   QRS
   QRST
   QS_1
   QS_2
   QT
   QTc
   QU
   Q to first sound
   right ventricular systolic time (RVSTI)
   RP
   RR
   S_1S_2
   S_1S_3
   S_2OS (second sound to opening snap)
   S-QRS

interval (cont.)
  ST
  systolic time (STI)
  VA
  VH
interventricular (IV)
interventricular septal defect
interventricular septum
intima
intimal dissection
intimal flap
intimal hyperplasia
intimal proliferation
intimal tear
intra-aortic balloon assist
intra-aortic balloon counterpulsation
intra-aortic balloon pump (IABP)
intra-arterially
intra-atrial baffle operation
intra-atrial conduction defect
intra-atrial reentry
intra-Hisian AV block
intra-Hisian delay
intracardiac mass
intracardiac pressure in Doppler echocardiogram
intracardiac shunt
Intracath catheter
intracavitary clot formation
intracavitary pressure-electrogram dissociation
intramyocardial
intranodal block
intraoperative digital subtraction angiography (IDSA)
intraperitoneal migration of pacemaker
intrapleural implantation of pulse generator
intrapulmonary shunting
intraretinal microangiopathy (IRMA)
intravascular volume status
intravascularly volume depleted

intravenous (I.V.)
intravenous TKO (to keep open [the vein, needle, or catheter])
intraventricular block, conduction delay
intraventricular conduction defect
intraventricular conduction delay
intraventricular systolic tension
intrinsicoid deflection
introducer
  Check-Flo
  Desilets-Hoffman catheter
  electrode
  Hemaquet catheter
  Hemaquet sheath
  heparin lock
  Littleford-Spector
  LPS Peel-Away
  Mullins catheter
  peel-away
  percutaneous lead
  permanent lead
  Tuohy-Bost
intubate, intubation
inversion
inverted P wave
inverted T wave
inverted terminal T wave
inverted U wave
iodine-123 heptadecanoic acid radioactive tracer
iodine-125 radioisotope
iohexol contrast medium
Ionescu method of making a trileaflet valve
Ionescu-Shiley bioprosthetic valve
Ionescu-Shiley bovine pericardial valve
Ionescu-Shiley heart valve
Ionescu-Shiley low-profile prosthetic valve
Ionescu-Shiley pericardial xenograft valve
Ionescu-Shiley standard pericardial prosthetic valve

iopamidol contrast medium
Iopamiron contrast medium (310; 370)
iothalamate meglumine contrast medium
ioxaglate meglumine contrast medium
IPG (impedance plethysmography)
IPH (intraplaque hemorrhage)
IPPA (iodine-123 phenylpentadecanoic acid)
ipsilateral nonreversed greater saphenous vein bypass
IRBBB (incomplete right bundle branch block)
Irex Exemplar ultrasound
IRMA (intraretinal microangiopathy)
irregularity
  diffuse
  luminal
  pulse
irregularly irregular heart rhythm
irritability, myocardial
Isch (ischemia)
ischemia
  cardiac
  exercise-induced
  global myocardial
  ischemic
  myocardial
  nonlocalized
  peri-infarction
  regional myocardial
  regional transmural
  remote
  silent
  silent myocardial
  subendocardial
  transient myocardial
ischemic changes, persistence of
ischemic episode
ischemic heart disease syndrome
ischemic rest pain
ischemic segment (on echocardiogram)
ischemic ST segment changes
ischemic viable myocardium
ischemic zone
ischemically mediated mitral regurgitation
isoelectric at J point
isoelectric line
isoelectric ST segment
isoenzyme
  cardiac
  CK
  CK-MB
  CK-MM
  CPK
  CPK-MB
  CPK-MM
  LDH_1
  LDH_2
isolated heat perfusion of an extremity
isometric exercise test
ISON (isosorbide dinitrate)
isorhythmic AV dissociation
Isovue-300 contrast medium
Isovue-370 contrast medium
Isovue-M 300 contrast medium
isthmus of aorta
ITA (internal thoracic artery) graft
IV (interventricular) septum
I.V. (intravenous)
I.V. bolus
I.V. drip
I.V. TKO (to keep open)
IVB (intraventricular block)
IVC (inferior vena cava)
Ivemark syndrome
IVS (interventricular septum)
IVSD (interventricular septal defect)
IVST (interventricular septal thickness)
Ivy bleeding time

J

J guide, Teflon
J guide wire
J junction on EKG
J loop technique on catheterization
J orthogonal electrode
J point on EKG
J tip wire
J tipped exchange guide wire
J wave on EKG
J wire
Jaccoud sign
jacket, Medtronic cardiac cooling
Jacobson-Potts clamp
Jahnke anastomosis clamp
Jako anterior commissure scope
James atrionodal bypass tract
James bundles or fibers
James intranodal bypass tract
Janeway lesion in infective endocarditis
Jannetta dissector
Jantene operation
Jarvik 7 (and 8) artificial heart
Jarvik 7-70 total artificial heart
Jatene-Macchi prosthetic valve
Javid carotid artery clamp
Javid endarterectomy shunt
jeopardy, myocardial
Jervell and Lange-Nielsen syndrome
JL4, JR4 (Judkins left [or right] 4 cm catheter
JL5, JR5 (Judkins left [or right] 5 cm catheter
Jobst compression stockings
Jobst-Stride support stockings
Jobst-Stridette support stockings
Johns Hopkins coarctation clamp
Johns Hopkins forceps
Johnson thoracic forceps
Jonas modification of Norwood procedure
Jones criteria for diagnosing acute rheumatic fever
Jones IMA forceps
Jones thoracic clamp
joule, joules
Judkins coronary catheter
Judkins cardiac catheterization
Judkins coronary arteriography
Judkins femoral catheterization
Judkins left coronary catheter
Judkins right coronary catheter
Judkins technique for coronary arteriography
Judkins USCI catheter
jugular venous distention (JVD)
jugular venous pressure (JVP)
jugular venous pulsation; pulse
jugulovenous distention (JVD)
Julian thoracic forceps
jump-graft
Junct (junctional)
junction
  aortic sinotubular
  atrioventricular
  J
  saphenofemoral
  sinotubular
junctional bradycardia
junctional escape beat
juxtapical impulse
JVD (jugulovenous or jugular venous distention)
JVP (jugular venous pressure)

K

kallikrein-kinin system
Kalos pacemaker
Kantrowitz vascular scissors
Kaposi sarcoma, epicardial
Kapp-Beck clamp
Kapp-Beck-Thomson clamp
Karmody venous scissors
Karp aortic punch forceps
Kartagener syndrome
Kartchner carotid artery clamp
Kasabach-Merritt syndrome
Kastec mitral valve prosthesis
Kattus treadmill exercise protocol
Katz-Wachtle phenomenon
Kawasaki syndrome
Kay tricuspid valvuloplasty
Kay-Lambert clamp
Kay-Shiley disk valve prosthesis
Kay-Shiley mitral valve
Kay-Suzuki disk prosthetic valve
Kaye-Damus-Stansel operation
Keith-Flack sinoatrial node
Kelly hemostat; retractor
Kelvin 500 Sensor pacemaker
Kennedy area-length method
Kennedy method for calculating ejection fraction
Kensey atherectomy catheter
Kent atrioventricular bundle
Kent bundles or fibers
Kerley A, B, or C lines
kick, atrial (AK)
Killip classification of heart disease
Killip classification of pump failure
Killip wire to give heart shock during cardiac arrest
Killip-Kimball classification of heart failure
kilopound
Kim-Ray Greenfield caval filter

Kindt carotid artery clamp
kinetocardiogram
King multipurpose coronary graft catheter
kinking of blood vessel
Kirklin atrial retractor
kissing balloon technique
Klein-Waardenburg syndrome
Klippel-Feil syndrome
knife
   Bailey-Glover-O'Neill commissurotomy
   Bard-Parker
   Beaver
   Brock commissurotomy
   cautery
   commissurotomy
   Derra commissurotomy
   intimectomy
   Lebsche sternal
knock, pericardial
Koch sinoatrial node
Koch, triangle of
Kono procedure for patch enlargement of ascending aorta
Kontron intra-aortic balloon
Korotkoff heart sound in blood pressure
Korotkoff method in Doppler cerebrovascular examination
Korotkoff test
Krayenbuehl vessel hook
Krehl, tendon of
Krovetz and Gessner equation
Kugel artery
Kugel anastomosis
Kugel collaterals
Kussmaul sign; syndrome
Kussmaul-Maier disease
KVO (keep vein open) rate

L

LA (left atrium)
LAA (left atrial appendage)
laboratory
  cardiac catheterization
  EP (electrophysiology)
L-transposition of great arteries
LACD (left apexcardiogram, calibrated displacement)
lactate dehydrogenase (LDH)
LAD (left axis deviation)
LAD (left anterior descending) artery
LAD wraps around the apex
LAD saphenous vein graft angioplasty
LAE (left atrial enlargement)
LAFB (left anterior fascicular block)
Lahey thoracic forceps
LAID (left anterior internal diameter)
Lambda pacemaker
Lambert aortic clamp
Lambert-Kay vascular clamp
Lambl excrescence
laminar flow
Lancisi sign
Landolfi sign
LAO (left anterior oblique) position; projection
LAP (left atrial pressure)
Laplace law; mechanism
laser
  argon
  CO_2 (carbon dioxide)
  Excimer
  helium-neon
  ion
  Nd:YAG
Laserdish electrode
Laserdish pacing lead
Laserprobe-PLR Plus

LASH (left anterior-superior hemiblock)
Lastac
late potential activity, ventricular
late systolic posterior displacement on echocardiogram
Laurence-Moon-Biedl syndrome
lavage
  bronchoalveolar (BAL)
  continuous pericardial
  pleural
  tracheal bronchial
law
  Einthoven
  Laplace
  Starling
LBBB (left bundle branch block)
LBCD (left border of cardiac dullness)
LCA (left coronary artery)
LCF or LCX (left circumflex) coronary artery
LDH (lactate dehydrogenase)
LDH_1 flip; isoenzyme
LDH_2 isoenzyme
LDL (low-density lipoprotein)
lead (see also *electrode*)
  I, II, III
  Accufix bipolar
  Accufix pacemaker
  Accufix pacing
  active fixation
  anterior precordial
  anterolateral
  anteroseptal
  atrial
  atrial J
  augmented EKG
  aV_F (aVF)
  aV_L (aVL)
  aV_R (aVR)
  barb-tip

| lead | 86 | leaflet |

lead *(cont.)*
  bipolar limb
  bipolar precordial
  break in insulation of
  chest
  CM_5
  cobra-head epicardial
  Cordis pacing
  CPI Sweet Tip
  dislodgement of
  EKG
  Encor pacing
  Endotak-C
  epicardial pacemaker
  esophageal
  finned pacemaker
  fishhook
  Frank XYZ orthogonal
  Hombach placement of
  impedance
  inferior
  inferior precordial
  inferolateral
  Laserdish pacing
  lateral
  lateral precordial
  left precordial
  Lewis
  limb
  Mason-Likar placement of EKG
  monitor
  orthogonal Frank XYZ EKG
  Oscor pacing
  pacemaker
  pacing
  precordial
  precordial EKG
  reversed arm
  right precordial
  right-sided chest
  scalar
  screw-on epicardial pacemaker
  screw-tipped
  silicone
  SRT (segmented ring tripolar)

lead *(cont.)*
  standard limb
  Telectronic pacing
  temporary pacemaker
  three-turn epicardial
  transvenous ventricular sensing
  two-turn epicardial
  unipolar limb
  unipolar precordial
  urethane
  ventricular
  $V_1 - V_6$
  Wilson central terminal on EKG
  XYZ Frank EKG
lead impedance
lead placement, chronic
lead reversal
lead threshold
leaflet, leaflets
  anterior mitral (AML)
  anterior motion of posterior
    mitral valve
  anterior tricuspid (ATL)
  aortic valve
  arching of mitral valve
  ballooning of
  billowing mitral (BML)
  bowing of mitral valve
  calcified
  cleft
  coaptation of
  degenerated
  doming of
  doughnut-shaped prolapsing
  flail mitral
  fluttering of valvular
  fused
  hammocking of
  incompetent
  mitral valve
  mural
  myxomatous valve
  nodularity of
  noncoronary
  paradoxical motion of

leaflet *(cont.)*
  poorly mobile
  posterior
  posterior mitral (PML)
  posterior tricuspid (PTL)
  prolapsed; prolapse of
  redundant
  retracted
  sail-like anterior
  septal
  thickened
  tricuspid valve
  valve
leaflet cleft
leaflet incompetence
leaflet motion
leaflet prolapse
  anterior
  posterior
leaflet tip
leak
  baffle
  interatrial baffle
  paraprosthetic
  paravalvular
  periprosthetic
  perivalvular
leaky valve
Leather valve cutter
Leather venous valvulotome
Lebsche sternal knife
Lectron II electrode gel
ledge, eccentric
Lee bronchus clamp
Lee microvascular clamp
Lee-White method
Lees artery forceps
left anterior descending (LAD) artery
left anterior fascicular block
left anterior hemiblock
left atrial appendage
left atrial enlargement
left axis deviation
left bundle branch block (LBBB)

left circumflex (LCX) coronary artery
left iliac system
left internal mammary artery (LIMA) graft
left sternal border
left-to-right shunt
left ventricular assist device (LVAD)
left ventricular dam
left ventricular end-diastolic pressure (LVEDP)
left ventricular end-diastolic volume
left ventricular end-systolic volume
left ventricular hypertrophy (LVH)
left ventricular regional wall motion
left ventricular segmental contraction
left ventricular systolic pump function
left ventricular systolic time interval ratio
leg fatigue
leg pain at rest
Legend pacemaker
Lehman ventriculography catheter
leiomyomatosis of heart
Leios pacemaker
Lejeune thoracic forceps
Leland-Jones vascular clamp
Lemmon intimal dissector
Lemmon sternal approximator
Lemmon sternal spreader
Lenegre disease
length
  basic cycle (BCL)
  basic drive (BDL)
  basic drive cycle (BDCL)
  chordal
  drive cycle
  paced cycle (PCL)
  sinus cycle
  VA block cycle
  wave
lentigines
lentiginosis, cardiomyopathic

Leptos-01 pacemaker
Leriche syndrome
lesion, lesions
  atherosclerotic
  bifurcation
  Blumenthal
  Bracht-Wachter
  calcified
  concentric
  coronary artery
  critical
  eccentric
  flow-limiting
  hemodynamically significant
  high-grade
  Janeway
  jet
  occlusive
  ostial
  partial
  regurgitant
  tandem
  tubular
  serial
  stenotic
  total
  vegetative
leukocyte-poor red blood cells
Leukos pacemaker
Lev classification of complete AV block
Lev disease; syndrome
LeVeen plaque-cracker
Levine sign
Levine-Harvey classification of heart murmur
levophase follow-through
levorotatory
levotransposition (L-transposition)
Lewis lead
Lewis and Pickering test
LGL (Lown-Ganong-Levine) variant syndrome
Libman-Sacks disease; syndrome

Libman-Sacks endocarditis
LICS (left intercostal space)
Liddle aorta clamp
lidocaine drip
Lido-Pen Auto-Injector
Liebermann-Burchard test
lifestyle, sedentary
lifestyle changes
lift
  aneurysmal
  late systolic parasternal
  left ventricular
  parasternal systolic
  pulmonary artery
  right ventricular
  substernal
  sustained right ventricular
ligament
  conus
  Cooper
ligamentum arteriosum
ligate, ligation
ligation, PDA (patent ductus arteriosus)
ligation of perforators
ligature
  rubber band
  silk
lightheaded
Lilienthal rib spreader
Lillehei valve forceps; prosthesis
Lillehei-Cruz-Kaster prosthesis
Lillehei-Kaster mitral valve prosthesis
Lillehei-Kaster pivoting-disk prosthetic valve
LIMA (left internal mammary artery) graft
limb, Gore-Tex
limb of bifurcation graft
Lincoln scissors
Lincoln-Metzenbaum scissors
Lindesmith operation
Lindholm tracheal tube

line
  A (arterial)
  anterior axillary
  aortic
  arterial
  central venous
  central venous pressure (CVP)
  commissural
  isoelectric
  Kerley A; B; C
  Linton
  midaxillary
  midclavicular (MCL)
  midsternal
  radial arterial
  suture
  venous
linea alba
lingular artery
Linton line
Linx exchange guide wire
Liotta total artificial heart
Liotta-BioImplant LPB prosthetic valve
lipemia retinalis
lipid
  plasma
  serum levels of
lipoprotein
  high-density (HDL)
  intermediate density (IDL)
  low-density (LDL)
  plasma
  very-low-density (VLDL)
lithium pacemaker
Littleford-Spector introducer
Littman defibrillation pad
Litwak cannula
Litwak left atrial-aortic bypass
Litwak mitral valve scissors
livedo reticularis
liver function
Livierato reflex
LMCA (left main coronary artery)
loading dose
lobe, sequestered (lung)
loculated collections of old clotted blood
Loeffler disease
Loeffler parietal fibroplastic endocarditis
long-axis parasternal view
Longdwel Teflon catheter
longitudinal arteriography
longitudinal incision
longitudinal narrowing
long QT syndrome
long segment narrowing
loop
  capillary
  endarterectomy
  Gerdy interauricular
  J (on catheterization)
  P
  QRS
  reentrant
  rubber vessel
  Silastic
  T
  vector
  ventricular
  vessel
Lo-Por vascular graft prosthesis
Lo-Pro tracheal tube
Lo-Profile and Lo-Profile II balloon catheter
Lo-Profile steerable dilatation catheter
loss of capture of pacemaker
loss of sensing of pacemaker
Louis, sternal angle of
Lovén reflex
low-amplitude P wave
low septal right atrium
low-density lipoprotein (LDL)
low-level treadmill
Lower-Shumway cardiac orthotopic transplant technique
Lown classification of ventricular premature beats

Lown modified grading system for ventricular arrhythmia
Lown-Ganong-Levine syndrome
LPA (left pulmonary artery)
LPFB (left posterior fascicular block)
LPH (left posterior hemiblock)
LPS balloon catheter
LPS Peel-Away introducer
LPV (left pulmonary vein)
LQTS (long QT syndrome)
LRA (low right atrium)
LSB (lower sternal border)
LSCVP (left subclavian central venous pressure)
L-transposition (levotransposition)
Lucchese mitral valve dilator
Luer fitting
Luer-Lok ports
Lumaguide catheter
lumen
  aortic
  vessel
luminal diameter
luminal irregularity
luminal narrowing
luminal stenosis
Lutembacher complex
Lutembacher syndrome
LV (left ventricular) function; pressure; wall motion
LVAD (left ventricular assist device)
LVAS (left ventricular assist system), Novacore
LVD (left ventricular dysfunction)
LVd (left ventricular diastolic dimension)
LVEDD (left ventricular end-diastolic dimension)
LVEDI (left ventricular end-diastolic volume index)
LVEDP (left ventricular end-diastolic pressure)
LVEF (left ventricular ejection fraction)
LVESD (left ventricular end-systolic dimension)
LVESVI (left ventricular end-systolic volume index)
LVET (left ventricular ejection time)
LVFS (left ventricular functional shortening)
LVFW (left ventricular free wall)
LVG (left ventriculogram)
LVH (left ventricular hypertrophy)
LVH with strain
LVID (left ventricular internal diameter or dimension)
LVIDD (left ventricular internal diastolic dimension)
LVIDd (left ventricular internal dimension at end-diastole)
LVIDs (left ventricular internal dimension at end-systole)
LVIV (left ventricular inflow volume)
LVM (left ventricular mass)
LVMI (left ventricular mass index)
LVOT (left ventricular outflow tract)
LVOV (left ventricular outflow volume)
LVP (left ventricular pressure)
LVP_1 and LVP_2 (left ventricular pressure on apex cardiogram)
LVPW (left ventricular posterior wall)
LVS (left ventricular systolic) pressure
LVs (left ventricular systolic) dimension
LVSW (left ventricular stroke work)
lytic intervention

M

m (meter; murmur)
M-mode Doppler echocardiography
M-mode echocardiogram
M-mode echophonocardiography
M-mode transducer
M pattern on right atrial waveform
M1 (marginal branch #1)
M$_1$ heart sound (mitral valve closure)
mA (milliampere)
MAC (mitral annular calcium)
MacCallum patch
machine
   Burdick EKG
   Cobe-Stockert heart-lung
   General Electric Pass-C echocardiograph
   Toshiba echocardiograph
macroangiopathy
Macrodex
Maestro pacemaker
magnet application over pulse generator
Magovern ball valve prosthesis
Magovern-Cromie ball-cage prosthetic valve
Mahaim bundles or fibers
Mahler sign
main pulmonary artery
major branches of coronary artery
maladie de Roger (Roger disease)
malaise
malar flush
malformation
   arteriovenous (AVM)
   coronary artery
Mallinckrodt angiographic catheter
malperfused, malperfusion
mammary souffle murmur
maneuver
   Adson
   costoclavicular

maneuver *(cont.)*
   hyperabduction
   Mueller
   Osler
   Rivero-Carvallo
   scalene
   squatting
   Valsalva
Mannkopf sign
manometer
   Riva-Rocci
   strain gauge
Mansfield balloon
Mansfield Scientific dilatation balloon catheter
manubrium
MAP (mean arterial pressure)
mapping
   activation-sequence
   body surface
   catheter
   Doppler color flow
   electrophysiologic
   endocardial catheter
   epicardial
   ice
   intramural
   precordial
   retrograde atrial activation
   sinus rhythm
marantic endocarditis
Marfan syndrome
marginal branch
marker, gold
marker-channel diagram
marker channel of pacemaker
markings, pulmonary vascular
Marquette 3-channel laser holder
Marshall, vein of
Martorell syndrome
Mary Allen Engle ventricle
Mason vascular clamp

Mason-Likar 12-lead ECG system
mass
   echogenic
   intracardiac
   intracavity
   intraventricular
   left ventricular (LVM)
   pulsatile abdominal
   right ventricular (RVM)
   ventricular
massage, carotid sinus
MAST (Medical Anti-Shock Trousers)
Master two-step exercise stress test
MAT (multifocal atrial tachycardia)
Matas aneurysmoplasty
Matson rib elevator; stripper
Matson-Alexander rib elevator
Mattox aorta clamp
maximum predicted heart rate (MPHR)
Maxon suture
Mayo exercise treadmill protocol
Mayo hemostat; scissors
Mayo ligature carrier
Mayo vein stripper
Mayo Pean forceps
MB band; fraction
MB isoenzyme of CK (CK-MB)
MBF (myocardial blood flow)
MBIH catheter
MCAT (myocardial contrast appearance time)
MCE (myocardial contrast echocardiography)
McGinn-White sign
McGoon coronary perfusion catheter
McHenry treadmill exercise protocol
mCi (millicurie)
McIntosh double-lumen catheter
MCL (midclavicular line)
MCS (middle coronary sinus)
MD-60 and MD-76 contrast medium

Meadox Microvel arterial graft
Meadox woven velour prosthesis
mean aortic pressure
mean arterial pressure (MAP)
mean cardiac vector
mean electrical axis
mean mitral valve gradient
mean rate of circumferential shortening
mean vectors
mechanism
   compensatory
   Frank Starling
   Laplace
   reserve
   sensing
   Starling
Medcor pacemaker
MEDDARS analysis system for cardiac catheterization
media (pl. of medium)
medication
   Abbokinase
   Abbokinase Open-Cath
   ACE (angiotensin-converting enzyme) inhibitor
   acebutolol
   acecainide
   acetazolamide
   Activase
   Adalat
   Adrenalin
   Adrin
   Alatone
   Alazide
   Alazine
   Aldactazide
   Aldactone
   Aldoclor
   Aldomet
   Aldoril
   alpha$_1$-adrenergic blocker agent
   alprostadil
   alteplase
   Amicar

medication (cont.)
  amiloride
  amiodarone
  amrinone lactate
  amyl nitrite
  angiotensin converting enzyme
    (ACE) inhibitors
  Anhydron
  anisindione
  anisoylated plasminogen strepto-
    kinase activator complex
    (APSAC)
  ansamycin (LM427)
  antiadrenergic agent
  antianginal agent
  antiarrhythmic agent
  anticoagulant
  antihyperlipidemic agent
  antihypertensive agent
  Aphrodyne
  Apresazide
  Apresodex
  Apresoline
  aprindine
  APSAC (anisoylated plasminogen
    streptokinase activator com-
    plex)
  AquaMephyton
  Aquatag
  Aquatensen
  Aramine
  Arfonad
  Arlidin
  Ascriptin
  aspirin
  atenolol
  Atromid-S
  atropine
  azathioprine
  Bantron
  batroxobin
  Baypress
  Benadryl
  bendroflumethiazide
  benzathine penicillin G

medication (cont.)
  benzthiazide
  bepridil
  beta blocker
  beta-adrenergic blocking agent
  betaxolol
  bicarb (sodium bicarbonate)
  Bicillin
  bile acid sequestrant
  Blocadren
  bretylium tosylate
  Bretylol
  Brevibloc
  bumetanide
  Bumex
  Calan
  Calciparine
  calcium antagonist
  calcium channel blocking agent
  calcium chloride
  calcium dobesilate
  Cam-ap-es
  Capoten
  Capozide
  captopril
  Cardene
  cardiac glycoside
  Cardilate
  Cardi-Omega 3
  Cardioquin
  cardioselective agent
  cardioselective beta blocker
  Cardizem SR
  Carfin
  Carwin
  Catapres
  Catapres-TTS-1; TTS-2; TTS-3
  Cedilanid-D
  Cerespan
  Cerubidine
  chlorothiazide
  chlorthalidone
  cholestyramine
  Choloxin
  Cholybar

medication *(cont.)*
chronotropic agent
cifenline succinate
Cin-Quin
Cipralan
CI-930
clofibrate
clonidine
Colestid
colestipol
Combipres
Cordarone
Corgard
Corzide
Coumadin
Crystodigin
Cyclan
cyclandelate
Cyclospasmol
cyclosporine
cyclothiazide
Demerol
Deponit
deslanoside
desmopressin acetate
dextrothyroxine
Diachlor
Diamox
diazoxide
dicumarol
digitalis
digitoxin
digoxin
Dilatrate-SR
dilevalol
diltiazem
dipyridamole
disopyramide
Diucardin
Diulo
Diupres
Diurese-R
Diuril
Diutensen-R
dobutamine

medication *(cont.)*
Dobutrex
Dopacard
dopamine
Dopastat
dopexamine
d-sotalol
Duotrate
Duraquin
Dyazide
Dyrenium
Ecotrin
Edecrin
edrophonium
eicosapentaenoic acid (EPA)
enalapril maleate
encainide
Enduron
Enduronyl Forte
Enkaid
enoximone
EPA (eicosapentaenoic acid)
ephedrine
epinephrine
ergonovine maleate
Ergotrate
erythrityl tetranitrate
Esidrix
Esimil
esmolol
ethacrynic acid
Ethaquin
Ethatab
ethaverine
Ethavex-100
Ethmozine
Ethon
Eutonyl Filmtabs
Eutron
Exna
felodipine
fish oil
flecainide
flosequinan
Fumide

medication *(cont.)*
 furosemide
 gemfibrozil
 Genabid
 guanabenz
 guanadrel
 guanethidine
 guanfacine
 Harmonyl
 HCTZ (hydrochlorothiazide)
 Healthbreak chewing gum
 heparin
 Hep-Lock
 HMG CoA reductase inhibitor
 Hydralazide
 hydralazine
 Hydrazide
 Hydrex
 hydrochlorothiazide (HCTZ)
 HydroDiuril
 hydroflumethiazide
 Hydromox R
 Hydropine
 Hydropres
 Hydrotensin
 Hydro-T
 Hygroton
 Hylidone
 Hylorel
 Hyperstat
 Hytrin
 indapamide
 Inderal
 Inderal LA
 Inderide LA
 Indocin
 indomethacin
 Inocor
 inotropic agent
 Intropin
 Inversine
 ISDN (isosorbide dinitrate)
 Ismelin
 Iso-Bid
 ISON (isosorbide dinitrate)

medication *(cont.)*
 Isonate
 isoproterenol
 Isoptin
 Isordil Tembids
 Isordil Titradose
 isosorbide dinitrate (ISDN)
 Isotrate Timecelles
 Isovex
 isoxsuprine
 Isuprel
 Kabikinase
 Klavikordal
 Konakion
 labetalol
 Lanoxicaps
 Lanoxin
 Lasix
 levarterenol
 Levophed
 lidocaine
 LidoPen Auto-Injector
 lignocaine
 Lipo-Nicin
 lisinopril
 lobeline
 Loniten
 loop diuretic
 Lopid
 Lopressor HCT
 Lorelco
 lovastatin
 Lozol
 Luramide
 Marazide
 Maxzide
 MDL-17043
 mecamylamine
 mephentermine
 Mephyton
 Metahydrin
 metaraminol
 Metatensin
 methoxamine
 methyclothiazide

medication (cont.)
    methyldopa
    metolazone
    metoprolol
    Mevacor
    mexiletine
    Mexitil
    Micro-K
    Microx
    Mictrin
    Midamor
    midodrine
    milrinone
    Minipress
    Minizide
    Minodyl
    minoxidil
    Miradon
    Moderil
    Moduretic
    morphine sulfate
    MS (morphine sulfate)
    n-3 fatty acids
    nadolol
    Napa
    Napamide
    Naptrate
    Naqua
    Naturetin
    Neo-Synephrine
    niacin
    Niazide
    Nicorette chewing gum
    nicotinic acid
    nifedipine
    nimodipine
    Nimotop
    Nipride
    nitrate, long-acting
    nitrates
    nitrendipine
    Nitro-Bid Plateau Caps
    Nitrocap T.D.
    Nitrocine Timecaps
    Nitrodisc

medication (cont.)
    Nitro-Dur II
    Nitrogard
    nitroglycerin (NTG)
    nitroglycerin spray
    Nitroglyn
    Nitrol
    Nitrol Patch
    Nitrolin
    Nitrolingual
    Nitronet
    Nitrong
    Nitropress
    nitroprusside
    Nitrospan
    Nitrostat
    nonselective beta blocker
    norepinephrine
    Normodyne
    Normozide
    Norpace CR
    NTG (nitroglycerin)
    Nylidrin
    Omega-3 fatty acid
    OPC-8212
    Oretic
    Oreticyl Forte
    Panwarfin
    papaverine
    pargyline
    Pavabid HP Capsulet
    Pavabid Plateau Caps
    Pavacap Unicelles
    Pavacen Cenules
    Pavadur
    Pavagen
    Pava-Par
    Pavarine Spancaps
    Pavased
    Pavasule
    Pavatine
    Pavatym
    Paverolan Lanacaps
    PDE isoenzyme inhibitor
    penicillin V

medication *(cont.)*
 pentaerythritol tetranitrate
 pentoxifylline
 Pentritol Tempules
 Pentylan
 peripheral vasodilator
 Peritrate SA
 Persantine
 PETN (pentaerythritol tetranitrate)
 PGE$_1$
 phentolamine
 phenylephrine
 pinacidil
 Pindac
 pindolol
 Plegisol
 polythiazide
 potassium chloride
 potassium-sparing diuretic
 potassium-wasting diuretic
 prazosin
 Prinivil
 Priscoline
 Proaqua
 probucol
 procainamide
 Procamide SR
 Procan SR
 Procardia
 Promega
 Promine
 Pronestyl-SR
 propafenone
 propranolol
 Prostin VR Pediatric
 protamine sulfate
 Proto-Chol
 Pyridamole
 Questran
 Quinaglute Dura-Tabs
 Quinatime
 Quinidex Extentabs
 quinidine gluconate
 quinidine polygalacturonate

medication *(cont.)*
 Quinora
 Quin-Release
 Raudixin
 Rauval
 Rauwiloid
 rauwolfia derivative
 Regroton
 Renese-R
 Reserpine
 Rhythmin
 Rythmo 1
 Saluron
 Salutensin
 Sandimmune
 SDPS (protamine solution)
 Seconal
 Sectral
 Ser-Ap-Es
 Serpalan
 Serpasil
 Serpazide
 silver acetate chewing gum
 sodium bicarbonate
 Sofarin
 Solu-Medrol
 Sorbitrate
 Spironazide
 spironolactone
 Spirozide
 Streptase
 streptokinase
 sublingual nitroglycerin
 Synkayvite
 Tambocor
 Tenex
 Tenoretic
 Tenormin
 Tensilon
 terazosin
 Thalitone
 thiazide diuretic
 Thiuretic
 Thrombinar
 thrombin, topical

medication *(cont.)*
  thrombolytic agent
  Thrombostat
  Timolide
  timolol
  tissue plasminogen activator (tPA)
  tocainide
  tolazoline
  Tonocard
  tPA (tissue plasminogen activator)
  Trandate
  Transderm-Nitro
  transdermal nitroglycerin
  Trental
  triamterene
  Trichlorex
  trichlormethiazide
  Tridil
  trimethaphan camsylate
  Unipres
  urokinase
  Valium
  Vaseretic
  Vasodilan
  vasodilator, peripheral
  Vasotec
  Vasoxyl
  verapamil
  Versed
  Visken
  Voxsuprine
  warfarin
  Wyamine
  Wytensin
  xamoterol
  Xylocaine
  Yocon
  yohimbine
  Yohimex
  Zaroxolyn
  Zestril
medial incision
median sternotomy incision
mediastinal lymph node
mediastinitis
mediastinoscope
mediastinoscopy
mediastinotomy
mediastinum, widened
Medicon rib spreader
Medicon vascular and cardiac surgery instruments
Medigraphics 2000 analyzer
MediPort implanted vascular access device
Medi-Quet surgical tourniquet
Meditech balloon catheter
Meditech steerable system
Medrad contrast medium injector
Medtel pacemaker
Medtronic aortic punch
Medtronic balloon catheter
Medtronic bipolar electrode
Medtronic cardiac cooling jacket
Medtronic Cardioverter
Medtronic demand pulse generator
Medtronic electrode
Medtronic-Hall monocuspid tilting-disk valve
Medtronic-Hall valve prosthesis
Medtronic Interactive Tachycardia Terminating System
Medtronic Minix
Medtronic pacemaker
Medtronic prosthetic valve
Medtronic Radio-Frequency (RF) Receiver
Medtronic SPO 502 pacemaker
Medtronic Symbios pacemaker
megahertz (MHz)
melena
Melrose solution
Meltzer sign
membrane
  fenestrated
  Gore-Tex surgical
  pleuropericardial
  supramitral

membrane oxygenator
membrane potential
Ménière syndrome
mercury-in-Silastic strain gauge for blood flow determination
Meridian echocardiography
Mersilene suture
mesh-wrapping of aortic aneurysm, subtotal
mesothelioma of atrioventricular node
mesoversion of heart
MET (measurement of oxygen consumption/kilogram/minute)
Meta MV pacemaker
metabolism, myocardial
metal needle
meter (m)
meter per second (m/sec) velocity
method (see also *formula*)
   Anel
   Antyllus
   Brasdor
   direct Fick
   Dodge area-length
   downstream sampling
   Fick
   forward triangle
   Graupner
   Hatle valve area
   Hetzel forward triangle
   indicator dilution
   Kennedy ejection fraction
   Lee-White
   metrizamide contrast medium
   Orsi-Grocco
   Pachon
   Purmann
   pyramid ventricular volume
   Scarpa
   Shimazaki area-length
   Theden
   upstream sampling
   Wardrop
   Westergren

Metzenbaum scissors
Meyer vein stripper
MFAT (multifocal atrial tachycardia)
MHz (megahertz)
MI (mitral insufficiency; myocardial infarction or ischemia)
Michel aortic clamp
microaneurysm
microangiopathy, intraretinal (IRMA)
microbubbles
   carbon dioxide
   hydrogen peroxide
   oxygen
   Renografin-76
microcavitation
microcirculation
microglide
Micro-Guide catheter
Microknit vascular graft prosthesis
Microlith P pacemaker
micromanometer-tip catheter
microsphere, albumin
microsphere perfusion scintigraphy
Microthin P2 pacemaker
Micro-Tracer portable EKG
midcircumflex
midclavicular line (MCL)
mid-diastolic (or middiastolic)
mid-distal
midlateral course
midportion
midsternal area
midsystole
midsystolic closure of aortic valve
midsystolic notching of velocity spectrum
midzone
Mikros pacemaker
Mikro-tip angiocatheter
Millar catheter-tip transducer
Millar micromanometer catheter
Millar pigtail angiographic catheter
Miller-Senn retractor
mill-house murmur

milliampere (mA)
millicurie (mCi)
Milliknit vascular graft prosthesis
millimeters of mercury (mmHg)
millisecond (msec)
millivolt (mv)
Mills arteriotomy scissors
Mills valvulotome
Mills valvotome
Miltex rib spreader
Milton disease
Mini-Profile dilatation catheter, USCI
minuscule
Minix ST pacemaker
Minnesota classification of EKG
Minnesota criteria for high R waves
minute volume
MIRI (myocardial infarction recovery index)
mirror-image brachiocephalic branching
missing a beat
mitral annular calcification
mitral configuration of cardiac shadow on x-ray
mitral insufficiency
mitral valve, parachute
mitral valve billowing
mitral valve leaflet tip
mitral valve prolapse syndrome
mitral valve regurgitation
mitral valve regurgitation without prolapse
mitral valve septal separation
mitral valve stenosis
Mitroflow pericardial prosthetic valve
Mitrothin P2 pacemaker
Mitsubishi angioscope
Mitsubishi angioscopic catheter
Mixter forceps
Mixter right-angle clamp
MM band; fraction
mmHg (millimeters of mercury)

M-mode Doppler echocardiography
M-mode echophonocardiography
M-mode transducer
Mobitz I and II AV heart block
Mobitz I second-degree block
Mobitz II second-degree block
Mobitz type I on Wenckebach heart block
Mobin-Uddin umbrella filter
modality
  pacing
  therapeutic
mode
  A- (echocardiogram)
  AAI (noncompetitive atrial demand)
  AAI rate-responsive
  atrial-burst
  atrial triggered and ventricular inhibited
  atrioventricular dual-demand
  B- (ultrasound)
  bipolar pacing
  committed
  DDD (fully automatic, atrioventricular universal dual-chamber)
  demand pacemaker
  dual-demand pacing
  DVI
  fixed rate
  full-to-empty VAD
  inhibited pacing
  M- (echocardiogram)
  noncommitted
  pacing
  semicommitted
  sequential
  stimulation
  synchronous pacemaker
  triggered pacing
  underdrive
  unipolar pacing
  VVI (noncompetitive demand ventricular)

mode abandonment
modified Bruce protocol
Mondor disease
monitor
   Accucap CO_2/O_2
   Accucom cardiac output
   Accutorr
   ambulatory Holter
   Arrhythmia Net arrhythmia
   CA (cardiac-apnea)
   cardiac
   CardioDiary heart
   Commucor A+V Patient
   continuous Holter
   Dinamap
   electrocardiograph
   Holter
   Ohmeda 6200 CO_2
monitoring
   bedside
   continuous Holter
   hemodynamic
monitoring line
Monneret pulse
monofilament absorbable suture
monophasic contour of QRS complex
Monorail angioplasty catheter
Morgagni, foramen of
Morris aorta clamp
Morse sternal spreader
Morton Salt Substitute
Moschcowitz disease; test
motion
   anterior wall
   apical wall
   brisk wall
   cusp
   dyskinetic wall
   hypokinetic wall
   inferior wall
   leaflet
   left ventricular regional wall
   paradoxical
   paradoxical leaflet

motion *(cont.)*
   paradoxical septal
   posterior wall
   posterolateral
   regional wall
   regional hypokinetic wall
   segmental wall
   septal wall
   systolic anterior (SAM)
   ventricular wall
moyamoya cerebrovascular disease
Moynahan syndrome
MPA (main pulmonary artery)
MPAP (mean pulmonary artery pressure)
MPF catheter
MPHR (maximum predicted heart rate)
MPR (myocardial perfusion reserve)
MR (mitral regurgitation)
MRI (magnetic resonance imaging)
   FLASH (fast low-angle shot) cardiac
   GRASS (gradient recalled acquisition in steady state) cardiac
MS (mitral stenosis; morphine sulfate)
msec (millisecond)
M-shaped pattern of mitral valve
MTT (mean pulmonary transit time)
mu (12th Greek letter) rhythm
Mueller maneuver; sign
MUGA (multiple gated acquisition) blood pool radionuclide scan
MUGA scan, preoperative resting
Muller catheter guide
Muller pediatric clamp
Muller-Dammann pulmonary artery banding
Mullins blade technique for dilatation of patent foramen ovale
Mullins catheter introducer
Mullins modification of transseptal catheterization

Mullins transseptal blade and balloon atrial septostomy
Mullins transseptal catheter
Mullins transseptal sheath
Multicor Gamma pacemaker
Multicor II pacemaker
multicrystal gamma camera
multifocal PVCs (premature ventricular contractions)
multiform PVC
multiform ventricular complexes
multilesion angioplasty
Multilith pacemaker
Multi-Med triple-lumen infusion catheter
multiple chord, center line technique in echocardiogram
multiprogrammable pulse generator
multipurpose catheter
mural thrombus
murmur
  accidental
  amphoric
  anemic
  aneurysmal
  aortic diastolic
  aortic insufficiency
  apex
  apical
  apical diastolic
  arterial
  atriosystolic
  attrition
  Austin Flint
  basal
  basal diastolic
  bellows (blowing)
  blood
  blowing
  blubbery diastolic
  brain
  Cabot-Locke
  cardiac
  cardiopulmonary
  cardiorespiratory

murmur *(cont.)*
  Carey Coombs
  coarse
  Cole-Cecil
  continuous
  continuous rumbling
  cooing
  cooing-dove
  Coombs
  crescendo
  crescendo-decrescendo
  crescendo-decrescendo configuration
  crescendo presystolic
  Cruveilhier-Baumgarten
  decrescendo
  diamond-shaped
  diastolic
  diastolic flow
  diffusely radiating
  diminuendo
  Docke
  Duroziez
  dynamic
  early diastolic
  early systolic
  ejection
  endocardial
  extracardiac
  Flint
  Frantzel
  friction
  functional
  functional heart
  Gallavardin
  Gibson
  goose honk
  grade 1 to 6 or I to VI
  grade 1/6 or I/VI; 2/6 or II/VI; 1-2/6 or I-II/VI
  Graham Steell heart
  groaning
  Hamman
  harsh
  heart

murmur *(cont.)*
  hemic
  high
  high-frequency
  high-pitched
  Hodgkin-Key
  holodiastolic
  holosystolic
  holosystolic ejection
  honking
  hourglass
  humming
  humming-top
  incidental
  increased during inspiration
  innocent
  innocent systolic
  inorganic
  late apical systolic
  late diastolic
  late-peaking systolic
  late systolic
  left ventricular outflow
  Levine Harvey grading system for
  loud
  low-frequency
  low-pitched
  machine-like
  machinery
  mammary souffle
  mid-diastolic flow
  midsystolic
  mid-to-late diastolic
  millwheel
  mill-house
  mitral
  mitral click
  musical
  nun's venous hum
  obstructive
  organic
  outflow
  pansystolic
  pathologic

murmur *(cont.)*
  pericardial
  pleuropericardial
  prediastolic
  presystolic (PSM)
  presystolic crescendo
  protodiastolic
  pulmonary outflow
  pulmonary valve flow
  pulmonic radiating
  rasping
  regurgitant
  Roger
  rumbling
  rumbling diastolic
  scratchy
  sea gull (or sea-gull)
  seesaw (to-and-fro)
  soft
  Steell
  stenosal
  Still
  subclavicular
  systolic
  systolic ejection
  to-and-fro (seesaw)
  Traube
  tricuspid diastolic
  vascular
  venous
  waterwheel
  whooping
murmur at the apex and left sternal border
murmur grades, I to VI; 1 to 6
murmur radiating to apex of heart
murmur radiating to axilla
murmur radiating to neck
murmur radiating to sternal border
murmur, rub, or gallop
murmur transmitted to apex of heart
murmur transmitted to axilla
murmur transmitted to base of heart

murmur transmitted to carotids
murmur transmitted to neck
murmur with/without radiation
muscle
muscular bridging
Musset sign
Mustard atrial baffle repair
Mustard procedure for transposition of great vessels
mv (millivolt)
MV (mitral valve)
MVA (mitral valve area)
MVD (mitral valve dysfunction)
MVO (maximum venous outflow)
MVO (mitral valve opening or orifice)
MVO_2 (myocardial oxygen consumption)
MVP (mitral valve prolapse)
MVR (mitral valve replacement)
MWT (maximum walking time)
Myler catheter
myocardial blood flow (MBF)
myocardial blush
myocardial bridging
myocardial contrast appearance time (MCAT)
myocardial infarction, stuttering
myocardial insufficiency, Sternberg
myocardial ischemia
myocardial lactate extraction (%)
myocardial necrosis
myocardial oxygen consumption
myocardial oxygen demand
myocardial stiffness
myocardial straining
myocardial stunning
myocardial uptake of thallium
myocarditis
    acute bacterial
    acute isolated
    bacterial
    chronic
    diphtheritic
    eosinophilic

myocarditis *(cont.)*
    fibrous
    Fiedler
    fragmentation
    fungal
    giant cell
    granulomatous
    Histoplasma
    hypersensitivity
    idiopathic
    infectious
    interstitial
    lymphocytic
    neutrophilic
    parenchymatous
    rheumatic
    subepicardial
    toxic
    Trichinella
    tuberculoid; tuberculous
    viral
myocardium
    hypertrophied
    ischemic viable
    ischemic reperfused
    jeopardized
    noninfarcted
    nonperfused
    perfused
    reperfused
    stunned
    viable
myopectoral inhibition of pacemaker
myoplasty, sartorius
myxedema
myxoma
    atrial
    biatrial
    cardiac
    pedunculated
    vascular
    ventricular
myxomatous degeneration of valve
myxomatous valve leaflet

N

N-13 ammonia uptake on PET scan
N-acetylprocainamide (NAPA) level
Nabatoff vein stripper
nadir of QRS complex
nadir, protodiastolic
nail-to-nailbed angle (clubbing)
NAPA (N-acetylprocainamide) level
Narcomatic flowmeter
narrowing
  arterial
  atherosclerotic
  diffuse
  focal
  high-grade
  residual luminal
  subcritical
nasal flaring
Nathan pacemaker
National Heart, Lung, and Blood
  Registry guidelines
National Institutes of Health (NIH)
  catheter
native coronary artery
native valve
native ventricle
native vessel
Naughton exercise test protocol
Naughton treadmill protocol,
  modified
Naughton-Balke treadmill protocol,
  modified
NBTE (nonbacterial thrombotic
  endocarditis)
Nd:YAG laser
near-syncopal episode
near syncope
neck of the aneurysm
neck veins
  distended
  flat
  fullness of

necrosis
  arteriolar
  coagulation
  cystic medial
  embolic
  Erdheim cystic medial
  myocardial
necrotizing arterial disease
needle
  AMC
  aortic root perfusion
  Becton Dickinson Teflon-
    sheathed
  Bengash-type
  Brockenbrough
  BV-2
  cardioplegic
  Cope biopsy
  Cournand
  cutting
  DLP cardioplegic
  large-bore
  metal
  Nordenstrom (Rotex II) biopsy
  pericardiocentesis
  Potts
  root
  Rotex II biopsy
  spinal
  swaged-on
  THI
  venting aortic Bengash-type
needle holder
  Berry sternal
  Vital Cooley microvascular
  Vital Ryder microvascular
needle, sponge, and instrument
  counts
NEFA (non-esterified fatty acid)
  scintigraphy
negative deflection on EKG

Nelson scissors
Nelson thoracic trocar
neoaorta
Neos 01-28 pacemaker
Neos M pacemaker
nephrosclerosis
nerve of Hering
nerve of Kuntz
NESC (nonejection systolic click)
New York Heart Association (NYHA) classification of angina
Newman-Keuls test
NH region of AV node
Nicolet CA100 apparatus for visual evoked potential
nidus
Niedner anastomosis clamp
night sweats
NIH left ventriculography catheter
NIH mitral valve forceps
nipple, blind
nitrate
NI-NR (no infection–no rejection)
nitroglycerin (NTG)
    sublingual (SL)
    topical
    transdermal
    translingual
    transmucosal
nitroglycerin drip
nl, Nml (normal)
nociceptive
nodal escape
nodal premature contraction
nodal rhythm
node
  aortic window
  Aschoff
  Aschoff-Tawara
  atrioventricular (AV, AVN)
  axillary lymph
  Flack
  Keith-Flack sinoatrial
  Koch sinoatrial
  lymph

node *(cont.)*
  mediastinal lymph
  NH region of AV
  Osler
  pericardial lymph
  SA (sinoatrial)
  shotty lymph
  sinoatrial (SA, SAN)
  sinus
  supraclavicular lymph
  Tawara atrioventricular
nodoventricular bypass fiber; tract
nodoventricular pathway
nodoventricular tachycardia
nodularity of valve leaflet
nodule
  Albini
  aortic valve
  Arantius
  Aschoff
  Bianchi
  Cruveilhier
  Kerckring
  Morgagni
  ossific
noncompensatory pause
noncoronary sinus
noncrushing vascular clamps
nondecremental
nondominant vessel
nondrinker, nonsmoker
nonejection systolic click (NESC)
noneverting suture
noninfarcted segment
noninvasive assessment
noninvasive technique
noninvasive testing
non-lifestyle-limiting lower extremity claudication
nonoperable disease
non-Q wave
nonselective beta blocker
nonsmoker, nondrinker
nonspecific changes
nonspecific ST segment changes

nonspecific ST and T wave changes
    (NSTTWC)
nonspecific T wave abnormality
nonspecific T wave aberration
nonspecific T wave changes
nontransmural myocardial infarction
nonvalved conduit
nonviable scar from myocardial
    infarction
Noon AV fistula clamp
Noonan syndrome
Nordenstrom biopsy needle
normal (nl, Nml)
normal S_1 and S_2
normal sinus rhythm (NSR)
normalization of inverted T waves
normotensive
normothermia
Norwood procedure
    Fontan modification of
    Gill-Jonas modification of
    hypoplastic left-sided heart
    Jonas modification of
    Sade modification of
    univentricular heart
NOS (not otherwise specified)
NoSalt
notch
    anacrotic
    aortic
    dicrotic
    sternal
    suprasternal

notched P wave
notching of pulmonic valve on
    echocardiogram
Nova II pacemaker
Nova MR pacemaker
Novacore LVAS (left ventricular
    assist system)
Novofil suture
NPC (nodal premature contraction)
NPJT (nonparoxysmal AV junc-
    tional tachycardia)
NPRJT (nonparoxysmal recipro-
    cating junctional tachycardia)
NSR (normal sinus rhythm)
NSTTWC (nonspecific ST and
    T wave changes)
NTG (nitroglycerin)
NTP (noninvasive temporary pace-
    maker)
null point
nun's murmur (venous hum)
Nurolon suture
Nu-Salt
nutrient cardioplegia
Nycore angiography catheter
NYHA (New York Heart Associa-
    tion)
NYHA classification of angina
NYHA classification of congestive
    heart failure
Nyquist limit

O

O point of cardiac apex pulse
O_2 carrying capacity
O_2 consumption index
O_2 extraction
O_2 via nasal cannula
oat bran
obliquity
obstruction
   aortic outflow
   congenital left-sided outflow
   cowl-shaped
   fixed coronary
   preocclusive
   pulmonary outflow
   subvalvular diffuse muscular
obstructive mitral valve murmur
obstructive murmur
obturator
obtuse marginal artery; branch
occlude, occluded
occluder
   Flo-Rester vessel
   Hunter-Sessions balloon
   radiolucent plastic
occlusion
   complete
   coronary
   embolic
   graft
   pressure-controlled intermittent coronary (PICSO)
   subtotal
   total
Ochsner forceps
Ochsner retractor
ocular pneumoplethysmography (OPG)
oculoplethysmography/carotid phonoangiography (OPG/CPA)
ODAM defibrillator
OHD (organic heart disease)

Ohmeda 6200 CO_2 monitor
oligemia
Olympus angioscope
OMB (obtuse marginal branch)
OMB1 (obtuse marginal branch #1)
Omnicarbon prosthetic valve
Omnicor pacemaker
Omniflex balloon catheter
Omni-Orthocor II pacemaker
Omnipaque contrast medium
Omniscience prosthetic valve
Omniscience tilting-disk valve prosthesis
Omni-Stanicor pacemaker
Omni-Theta pacemaker
O'Neill clamp
OPC (ophthalmoplethysmography)
opening
   amplitude of valve
   valvular
opening snap (OS)
operation
   ablation of bundle of His
   aneurysmectomy
   annuloplasty
   aortic root replacement
   aortic valve replacement
   aortic valvuloplasty
   aortofemoral bypass
   aortopulmonary window
   arterial switch
   arteriotomy
   atherectomy
   atrial baffle
   atrioventricular valve replacement
   AV (aortic valve) repair
   balloon atrial septostomy
   balloon mitral valvuloplasty
   balloon valvuloplasty
   banding of pulmonary artery
   Bentall inclusion technique

operation *(cont.)*
  BIMA (bilateral internal mammary artery) reconstruction
  blade and balloon atrial septostomy
  Blalock-Hanlon atrial septectomy
  Blalock-Taussig anastomosis
  Brockenbrough commissurotomy
  CABS (coronary artery bypass surgery)
  Carpentier annuloplasty
  Carpentier tricuspid valvuloplasty
  catheter ablation of bundle of His
  catheter balloon valvuloplasty (CBV)
  coarctectomy
  commissurotomy
  Cooley anastomosis
  cryosurgery
  cryosurgical interruption of AV node; bypass tract
  De Vega annuloplasty
  division of accessory bundle of Kent
  electrode catheter ablation
  encircling endocardial ventriculotomy
  endocardial to epicardial resection
  femorodistal bypass
  femoropopliteal bypass
  Fontan tricuspid atresia
  Fontan-Kreutzer repair
  Glenn
  heart transplant
  heart-lung transplant
  Hunter
  infarctectomy
  inferior vena cava interruption
  infundibular resection
  intra-atrial baffle
  Jantene

operation *(cont.)*
  Kay tricuspid valvuloplasty
  Kaye-Damus-Stansel
  Kono
  laser recanalization
  Lindesmith
  Lower-Shumway heart transplant
  Matas aneurysmoplasty
  median sternotomy
  mitral valve replacement
  Muller-Dammann pulmonary artery banding
  Mullins blade and balloon septostomy
  Mullins transseptal atrial septostomy
  Mustard atrial baffle repair
  Mustard transposition of great arteries
  Norwood hypoplastic left-sided heart
  Norwood univentricular heart procedure
  open heart
  open mitral commissurotomy
  orthotopic cardiac transplant
  palliative
  Park blade and balloon atrial septostomy
  patent ductus arteriosus (PDA) ligation
  percutaneous aortic valvuloplasty (PAV)
  percutaneous mitral balloon valvotomy (PMV)
  percutaneous transluminal balloon dilatation (PTBD)
  pericardiectomy
  peripheral artery bypass
  peripheral laser angioplasty (PLA)
  phlebectomy
  photoablation, laser
  plication repair of flail leaflet

operation *(cont.)*
   postcardiotomy intra-aortic balloon pumping
   Potts-Smith side-to-side anastomosis
   profunda Dacron patchplasty
   profundaplasty
   pulmonary artery banding
   pulmonary balloon valvuloplasty
   pulmonary valvotomy
   pulmonary valvuloplasty
   Rashkind-Miller atrial septostomy
   Rastelli
   recanalization
   redirection of inferior vena cava
   Reed ventriculorrhaphy
   Sade modification of Norwood
   sandwich patch closure
   Schede thoracoplasty
   selective subendocardial resection
   Senning atrial baffle repair
   Senning transposition
   septectomy
   septostomy
   SIMA (single internal mammary artery) reconstruction
   Simpson atherectomy
   stellectomy
   Sucquet-Hoyer anastomosis
   Sugiura esophageal varices
   sympathectomy, regional cardiac
   systemic to pulmonary artery anastomosis
   thromboendarterectomy
   thrombolysis, intracoronary
   transcatheter closure of atrial septal defect
   triangular resection of leaflet
   tricuspid valve annuloplasty
   transmural resection
   valvotomy
   valvuloplasty
   valvulotomy
   vein stripping

operation *(cont.)*
   venotomy
   ventricular exclusion
   ventriculorrhaphy
   ventriculotomy
   Waterston extrapericardial anastomosis
   wedge-shaped sleeve aneurysm resection
   wrapping of abdominal aortic aneurysm
OPG (oculo- or ophthalmoplethysmography)
OPG/CPA (oculoplethysmography/carotid phonoangiography)
Op-Site dressing
Optima MP pacemaker
Optima MPI Series III pulse generator
Optima MPT Series III pacemaker
Optima SPT pacemaker
Optiscope catheter
orifice
   atrioventricular
   cardiac
   coronary
   double coronary
   narrowed
   valve
origin of artery
Orion pacemaker
Orsi-Grocco method
ORT (orthodromic reciprocating tachycardia)
Orthocor II pacemaker
orthodromic AV reciprocating tachycardia
orthodromic reciprocating tachycardia (ORT)
orthogonal lead arrangement for EKG
orthopnea
   three-pillow
   two-pillow

orthostasis
orthostatic blood pressure
orthostatic hypotension
orthostatism, vasovagal
os, coronary
OS (opening snap)
Osborn wave on EKG
oscillatory
oscilloscope, Tektronix
Oscor active fixation leads
Oscor pacing lead
O'Shaughnessy artery forceps
Osler maneuver; node; sign
osteomyelitis of sternum
osteosarcoma of heart
ostia of artery
ostial cannulation
ostium, ostia
   aortic
   coronary
ostium primum defect
ostium secundum defect
outflow anastomosis
outflow, maximum venous (MVO)
outflow tract
output
   cardiac (CO)
   Dow method for cardiac
   Fick method for cardiac
   Gorlin method for cardiac
   Hetzel forward triangle method for cardiac
   pulmonic
   Stewart-Hamilton technique for cardiac
   stroke
   systemic
   thermodilution cardiac
   ventricular
overdrive pacing
overdrive suppression
Overholt thoracic forceps
overload, overloading
   right ventricular
   systolic ventricular volume
overriding of aorta
oversensing, pacemaker
Owren disease
oximeter
   American Optical ear
   Hewlett-Packard ear
   intracardiac
oximetry
   ear
   reflectance
Oxycel
oxygen by nasal cannula
oxygen capacity
oxygen consumption, increased
oxygen content
oxygen extraction
oxygen saturation (%)
oxygen stepup (or step-up)
oxygenated blood
oxygenation, extracorporeal membrane
oxygenator
   Bentley
   bubble
   Capiox-E bypass system
   disk
   film
   membrane
   pump
   rotating disk
   screen
   Shiley
oxyhemoglobin dissociation curve

P

P (posterior)
P₂T₀ interval
P₂ heart sound (pulmonary valve closure)
P cell
P congenitale
P loop
P mitrale
P pulmonale in leads II, III, aV_F
P pulmonale syndrome
P terminal force abnormality
P synchronous pacing
P vector
P wave
  bifid
  biphasic
  depressed
  diphasic
  flattened
  inverted
  low-amplitude
  nonconducted
  notched
  peaked
  pointed
  retrograde
  tall
  terminal negativity of
  upright
  widened
P wave amplitude
PA (pulmonary artery) pressure
PA diastolic pressure
PA interval
PA systolic pressure
PAB (premature atrial beat)
PABP (pulmonary artery balloon pump)
PAC (premature atrial complex or contraction)
paced impulse
paced ventricular evoked response (PVER)
pacemaker, cardiac (see also *generator*)
  AAI (atrial demand inhibited)
  AAT (atrial demand triggered)
  Accufix
  Acculith
  Activitrax
  Activitrax II single-chamber VVI
  Activitrax variable rate
  activity sensing
  Aequitron
  AFP
  AICD
  AID-B
  AOO (atrial asynchronous)
  Arco
  Arcolithium
  artificial
  Arzco
  Astra
  ASVIP (atrial synchronous, ventricular inhibited)
  asynchronous mode
  atrial synchronous, ventricular-inhibited (ASVIP)
  atrial tracking
  atrial triggered, ventricular inhibited
  Atricor
  atrioventricular sequential
  Aurora dual-chamber
  Autima II dual-chamber cardiac
  AV junctional
  AV sequential
  Avius sequential
  Basix
  Biotronik
  bipolar
  burst

pacemaker *(cont.)*
  Byrel SX
  Byrel-SX/Versatrax
  Cardio-Pace Medical Durapulse
  Chardack-Greatbatch implantable cardiac pulse generator
  Chorus
  Chronocor IV external
  Classix
  Command PS
  committed mode
  Cook
  Cordis
  Cordis Gemini
  Cordis Sequicor
  Cosmos pulse generator
  Cosmos II DDD
  Cosmos 283 DDD
  CPI (Cardiac Pacemakers, Inc.)
  CPI Astra
  CPI 910 ULTRA II
  cross-talk
  Cyberlith
  Cybertach 60
  Cybertach automatic-burst atrial
  Daig ESI-II or DSI-III screw-in lead
  DDD (fully automatic sequential)
  DDI mode
  Delta
  demand
  Devices, Ltd.
  Diplos M
  downward displacement of
  dual-chamber
  Durapulse
  DVI (AV sequential)
  Ectocor
  ectopic atrial
  Ela
  Electrodyne
  Elema-Schonander
  Elevath
  Elgiloy
  Encor

pacemaker *(cont.)*
  Enertrax
  external transthoracic
  externally controlled noninvasive programmed stimulation
  Fast-Pass lead
  fixed rate, asynchronous atrial
  fixed rate, asynchronous ventricular
  fully automatic, atrioventricular universal dual-channel
  Galaxy
  Gemini 415 DDD
  General Electric
  Genisis *(not* Genesis)
  Guardian
  hermetically sealed standby
  Intermedics
  Intermedics Quantum
  Intertach 262-12
  intraperitoneal migration of
  junctional
  Kalos
  Kelvin 500 Sensor
  Lambda
  latent
  Legend
  Leios
  Leptos-01
  Leukos
  lithium
  loss of capture in
  Maestro
  Medcor
  Medtel
  Medtronic
  Medtronic RF 5998
  Medtronic SPO 502
  Medtronic Symbios
  Meta MV
  Microlith P
  Midros
  Minix ST
  Mitrothin P2
  Multicor Gamma

pacemaker *(cont.)*
  Multicor II
  Multilith
  multiprogrammable
  myopectoral inhibition of
  Nathan
  Neos M; 01-28
  noncompetitive
    atrial demand
    atrial synchronous
    atrial triggered
    demand ventricular
    ventricular synchronous
    ventricular triggered
  noninvasive temporary (NTP)
  Nova MR; II
  Omnicor
  Omni-Orthocor
  Omni-Stanicor
  Omni-Theta
  Optima MPI Series III pulse generator
  Optima MP; MPT; SPT
  Orion
  Orthocor II
  oversensing
  Pacesetter
  Pacesetter AFP
  Pacesetter Synchrony
  Pacesetter systems
  PASAR (permanent scanning antitachycardia)
  PASAR tachycardia reversion
  Pasys
  permanent
  permanent rate-responsive
  permanent ventricular
  Permathane Pacesetter lead
  Phoenix single-chamber
  Pinnacle
  PolyFlex lead
  Prima
  Prism-CL
  Programalith
  programmable

pacemaker *(cont.)*
  Prolith
  Pulsar NI
  P wave triggered ventricular
  QT sensing
  Quantum
  radiofrequency
  rescuing
  respiratory-dependent
  RS4
  screw-in lead
  Seecor
  Sensolog
  Sensor Kelvin
  Sequicor
  Siemens-Elema
  Siemens-Pacesetter
  single-chamber
  sinus node
  Sorin
  Spectraflex
  Spectrax programmable Medtronic
  Spectrax SXT
  standby
  Stanicor
  Starr-Edwards
  Symbios
  synchronous mode
  Synergyst DDD
  tachycardia-terminating
  Tachylog
  Telectronics
  temporary
  temporary transvenous
  Thermos
  tined lead
  transcutaneous
  transthoracic
  transvenous
  Trios M
  troubleshooting of
  undersensing malfunction of
  Unilith
  unipolar

pacemaker *(cont.)*
  variable rate
  VAT (atrial synchronous ventricular)
  VDD (atrial synchronous ventricular inhibited)
  Ventak AICD
  Ventricor
  ventricular
  Versatrax and Versatrax II
  Vicor
  Vista
  Vitatrax II
  Vitatron
  VOO (ventricular asynchronous)
  VVI (ventricular demand inhibited)
  VVI/AAI
  VVT (ventricular demand triggered)
  wandering atrial (WAP)
  Xyrel
  Zitron
  Zoll NTP (noninvasive temporary)
pacemaker afterpotential
pacemaker amplifier refractory period
pacemaker amplifier sensitivity
pacemaker AV disable mechanism
pacemaker battery
pacemaker battery status
pacemaker burst pacing
pacemaker capability
pacemaker capture
  erratic
  lack of
pacemaker cell
pacemaker electrode
pacemaker escape interval
pacemaker failure
pacemaker generator pouch
pacemaker hysteresis
pacemaker implantation
pacemaker introducer

pacemaker lead
pacemaker lead impedance
pacemaker loss of capture
pacemaker loss of sensing
pacemaker malfunction
pacemaker marker channel
pacemaker oversensing
pacemaker pacing mode
pacemaker pocket
pacemaker programmability
pacemaker programmed settings
pacemaker rate
pacemaker reedswitch
pacemaker reprogramming
pacemaker sensing
pacemaker sensitivity
pacemaker spike
pacemaker stimulus output amplitude
pacemaker syndrome
pacemaker system analyzer
pacemaker tester system
pacemaker threshold
pacemaker undersensing
pacemapping
Paceport catheter
Pacesetter AFP pacemaker
Pacesetter cardiac pacemaker
Pacesetter Synchrony
Pacesetter systems pacemaker
Pachon method; test
pacing
  antitachycardia
  asynchronous
  asynchronous atrioventricular sequential
  atrial
  atrial overdrive
  atrial synchronous ventricular
  autodecremental
  AV sequential
  backup bradycardia
  burst-overdrive
  cardiac
  committed

pacing *(cont.)*
  competitive
  coronary sinus
  coupled
  demand
  double ventricular
  dual-chamber
  endocardial
  epicardial
  external
  external cardiac
  fixed rate
  incremental
  incremental atrial
  noncommitted
  overdrive
  paired
  permanent
  P synchronous
  P triggered ventricular
  rapid atrial
  rapid ventricular
  rate adaptive
  rate responsive (RRP)
  scanning
  semicommitted
  sequential
  synchronous
  temporary cardiac
  temporary transvenous
  transcutaneous
  transesophageal
  transesophageal atrial
  transesophageal cardiac
  transthoracic cardiac
  triggered
  ventricular
  ventricular cardiac
  ventricular demand
  ventricular overdrive
  ventricular triggered
  vibration based
pacing analyzer
pacing-induced termination of
  arrhythmia
pacing stimulus
pacing system analyzer (PSA)
pacing threshold
pacing wire
pacing wire fracture
pack, moist laparotomy (lap)
packed cells
pack-years of cigarette smoking
$PaCO_2$
pad
  defibrillator
  laparotomy (lap)
  Littmann defibrillation
  R-2
pad sign of aortic insufficiency
PAD (pulmonary artery diastolic)
  pressure
PAD (pulsatile assist device)
paddle, defibrillatory
PADP-PAWP (pulmonary artery
  diastolic and wedge pressure)
  gradient
PAEDP (pulmonary artery end-
  diastolic pressure)
pain (see also *angina*)
  anginal chest
  atypical chest
  burning
  calf
  chest
  crushing chest
  dull
  exertional chest
  focal
  ischemic rest
  pinching chest
  pleuritic
  precordial
  pressure
  radiating to left arm/shoulder
  referred cardiac
  rest
  retrosternal chest
  squeezing chest
  sternal border

pain *(cont.)*
   suffocating chest
palliation, palliative
palliative operative procedure
pallor, elevation
pallor of extremity
Palmaz vascular stent
palpation, precordial
palpitation(s)
   flip-flop
   flopping
   fluttering
PAM (pulmonary artery mean) pressure
PAN (periarteritis nodosa)
pancarditis
panchamber enlargement
pansystolic murmur
pantyhose, support (see *stockings*)
PaO₂
PAP (pulmonary artery pressure)
papillary muscle dysfunction
papillary muscle rupture
papilledema
PAPVR (partial anomalous pulmonary venous return)
parachute deformity of mitral valve
parachute mitral valve
paracorporeal
paradoxical motion
paradoxical pulse
paradoxical septal motion
parameter, physiologic
parameters, clinical
paraneoplastic syndrome; process
paraprosthetic leakage
paraseptal position
parasternal long-axis view
parasternal short-axis view
parasternal systolic lift
parasternal view of heart
parasystole
   atrial
   junctional
   ventricular

paravalvular
parietal pericardium
Park blade septostomy
Park blade and balloon atrial septostomy
Parks 800 bidirectional Doppler flowmeter
paroxysmal atrial tachycardia (PAT)
paroxysmal nocturnal dyspnea (PND)
paroxysmal nocturnal hemoglobinuria (PNH)
paroxysmal tachycardia
Parsonnet probe
partial anomalous pulmonary venous connection
partial anomalous pulmonary venous return (PAPVR)
partial occlusion clamp
parvus et tardus, pulsus
parvus pulse
PAS (pulmonary artery systolic) pressure
PASAR (permanent scanning antitachycardia) pacemaker
PASAR tachycardia reversion pacemaker
PASP/SASP (pulmonary to systemic arterial systolic pressure) ratio
passer
   right-angle
   Schmidt
PASYS (single-chamber cardiac pacing system)
Pasys pacemaker
PAT (paroxysmal atrial tachycardia)
PAT with block
patch
   autologous pericardial
   Carrel
   Dacron
   Dacron Sauvage
   felt
   Gore-Tex cardiovascular
   Gore-Tex soft tissue

patch *(cont.)*
  gusset-type
  MacCallum
  outflow cardiac
  pericardial
  Teflon
  Teflon felt
  Teflon intracardiac
  transannular
  transdermal nitroglycerin
patch closure of septal defect
patch-graft aortoplasty
patch-graft, Dacron onlay
patchplasty, profunda Dacron
patency, coronary bypass graft
patency of vein graft
patency of vessel
patent, widely
patent ductus arteriosus (PDA)
patent graft
Pathfinder catheter
pathway
  accessory (AP)
  accessory AV
  accessory conduction (ACP)
  antegrade
  anterior internodal
  atrioventricular
  atrio-His; atrio-Hisian
  AV nodal
  Bachmann
  bystander
  concealed accessory
  dual AV nodal
  free-wall accessory
  internodal
  nodoventricular
  paranodal
  paraseptal accessory
  posterior septal
  preferential intranodal
  reentrant
  retrograde
  septal
  Thorel

pathway *(cont.)*
  Wenckebach
pathways, multiple accessory
pattern
  A fib (atrial fibrillation)
  bigeminal
  blood flow
  contractile
  dP/dt upstroke
  early repolarization
  juvenile T wave
  left ventricular contraction
  left ventricular strain
  M (on right atrial waveform)
  M-shaped mitral valve
  pulmonary flow
  pulmonary vascular
  P pulmonale
  QR
  right ventricular strain
  RR' (RR prime)
  RSR' (RSR prime)
  S_1Q_3
  $S_1Q_3T_3$
  $S_1S_2S_3$
  speckled
  spectral
  strain
  trigeminal
  ventricular contraction
pause
  compensatory
  noncompensatory
  postextrasystolic
PAV (percutaneous aortic valvuloplasty)
PAWP (pulmonary artery wedge pressure)
PBF (pulmonary blood flow)
PBLs (peripheral blood lymphocytes)
PBPI (penile-brachial pressure index) to assess cardiac disease
PBVI (pulmonary blood volume index)

PCG (phonocardiogram)
PCL (paced cycle length)
pCO$_2$
PCP (pulmonary capillary pressure)
PCS (proximal coronary sinus)
PCVD (pulmonary collagen vascular disease)
PCWP (pulmonary capillary wedge pressure)
PDA (patent ductus arteriosus on echo report; posterior descending artery on cath report)
PDE isoenzyme inhibitor
PDS sutures
PDT guide wire
PE (pericardial effusion; pulmonary embolus)
peak and trough drug levels
peak circumferential wall stress
peak exercise
peak flow velocity
peak of wave
peak regurgitant flow velocity
peak systolic pressure
peak-to-peak pressure gradient
peak velocity of blood flow on Doppler echocardiogram
peaked P wave
Pean clamp
pectoralis fascia
pectoris, angina
pedal edema
pedal pulses, intact
pedicle
   IMA (internal mammary artery)
   phrenic
peel-away sheath
peeling back mechanism on electrophysiology study
PEEP (positive end-expiratory pressure)
PEI (postexercise index)
Pemco prosthetic valve
pencil, electrocautery
Penfield dissector
Penfield elevator
penicillin prophylaxis
penile-brachial pressure index (PBPI) to assess cardiac disease
Penn State total artificial heart
pentalogy, Fallot
PE Plus II balloon dilatation catheter
PEP (pre-ejection period)
percent of predicted maximum heart rate
Percor DL-II (dual-lumen) intraaortic balloon catheter
Percor-Stat-DL catheter
percussion wave of carotid arterial pulse
percutaneous groin puncture
percutaneous insertion
percutaneous intra-aortic balloon counterpulsation
percutaneous lead introducer
percutaneous puncture technique
percutaneous retrograde atherectomy
percutaneous transluminal angioplasty (PTA)
percutaneous transluminal coronary angioplasty (PTCA)
percutaneously cannulated
percutaneously inserted
percutaneously introduced
Perez sign
perforator (vessel), first septal
perforators
   ligation of
   stripping of
performance (see *function*)
perfusate
perfuse, perfused, perfusion
perfusion
   coronary
   extremity
   isolated heat
   myocardial
   peripheral

perfusion *(cont.)*
  pulsatile
  retrograde cardiac
  tissue
perfusion abnormality
perfusion defect
perfusion lung scan
perfusionist, pump
periaortic
periarteritis nodosa (PAN)
pericardial baffle
pericardial basket
pericardial cavity
pericardial disease
pericardial effusion with cardiac tamponade
pericardial flap
pericardial fluid
pericardial friction rub
pericardial knock
pericardial lavage, continuous
pericardial rub
pericardial sac
pericardial sinus
pericardial sling
pericardial space
pericardial tamponade
pericardiectomy
pericardiocentesis needle
pericardiotomy syndrome
pericarditis
  acute benign
  acute fibrinous
  adhesive
  amebic
  bacterial
  carcinomatous
  constrictive
  drug-induced
  dry
  effusion-constrictive
  external
  fibrinous
  hemorrhagic
  idiopathic

pericarditis *(cont.)*
  inflammatory
  localized
  mediastinal
  obliterating
  postinfarction
  postoperative
  purulent
  radiation-induced
  rheumatic
  serofibrinous
  Sternberg
  suppurative
  traumatic
  tuberculous
  uremic
  viral
pericarditis calculosa
pericarditis episternocardiaca
pericarditis obliterans
pericarditis sicca
pericarditis villosa
pericardium
  adherent
  bread-and-butter
  calcified
  diaphragmatic
  fibrous
  inflamed
  parietal
  pericardial
  shaggy
  visceral
peri-infarction block
peri-infarction conduction defect
peri-infarction ischemia
peri-infarctional defect
period
  absolute refractory (ARP)
  accessory pathway effective refractory
  antegrade refractory
  atrial effective refractory
  atrial refractory
  diastolic filling

period *(cont.)*
 effective refractory (ERP)
 ejection
 functional refractory (FRP)
 pacemaker amplifier refractory
 postventricular atrial refractory (PVARP)
 pre-ejection (PEP)
 presphygmic
 rapid filling (RFP)
 relative refractory (RRP)
 retrograde refractory
 sphygmic
 systolic ejection (SEP)
 ventricular effective refractory (VERP)
 ventriculoatrial effective refractory
 vulnerable
 Wenckebach
periodicity, AV node Wenckebach
periorbital Doppler study
periosteum, periosteal
peripelvic collateral vessel
peripheral blood lymphocytes (PBLs)
peripheral cyanosis
peripheral laser angioplasty (PLA)
peripheral pulse deficit
peripheral resistance
peripheral vascular disease, arteriosclerotic
periprosthetic leak
peritoneal dialysis, continuous ambulatory
perivalvular leak
Perma-Hand suture
permanent lead introducer
permanent rate-responsive pacemaker
Permathane Pacesetter lead pacemaker
peroneal-tibial trunk
personality type A; type B
Perthes test
pervenous catheter
PES (programmed electrical stimulation)
PET (positron emission tomography)
PET balloon with window and extended collection chamber
PET balloon, USCI
Pet balloon Simpson atherectomy device
PET scan
PETN (pentaerythritol tetranitrate)
PFD (persistent fetal dispersion) of AV node
PFR (peak filling rate)
PFWT (pain-free walking time) on treadmill
pH
PH interval
Phalen stress test
Phaneuf artery forceps
phase angle
phenomenon
 Aschner
 Ashman
 Austin Flint
 coronary steal
 dip
 embolic
 Gaertner
 Gallavardin
 gap conduction
 Goldblatt
 Katz-Wachtle
 R-on-T
 Raynaud
 Schellong-Strisower
 vasovagal
 Wenckebach
phlebectomy
phlebitis
phlebogram; -graphy
phleborheography
Phoenix single-chamber pacemaker
Phoenix total artificial heart
phonocardiogram (PCG)

phonocardiography, intracardiac
phonomechanocardiography
photic driving at select flash frequencies
photoablation, laser
photometer, HemoCue
phrenic nerve
phrenic pedicle
PHTN (pulmonary hypertension)
physiologic splitting of S_2
physiologic third heart sound
PI (pulmonic insufficiency)
PIB (peri-infarction block)
PIBC (percutaneous intra-aortic balloon counterpulsation)
PICA (posterior inferior communicating artery)
PICD (peri-infarction conduction defect)
Pick disease; syndrome
PICSO (pressure-controlled intermittent coronary occlusion)
Pierce-Donachy Thoratec VAD (ventricular assist device)
pigtail catheter
Pilling Wolvek sternal approximator
Pilotip catheter guide
pinching chest pain
pink tetralogy of Fallot
pinked up (verb)
Pinnacle pacemaker
PJC (premature junctional contraction)
PJT (paroxysmal junctional tachycardia)
PLA (peripheral laser angioplasty)
PLA-I (platelet antigen)
plane
  circular
  four-chamber
  frontal
  short-axis
  valve
planimeter, planimetry

plaque, plaquing (noun)
  arterial
  arteriosclerotic
  atheromatous
  atherosclerotic
  eccentric atherosclerotic
  fatty
  fibrous
  fibrotic
  fissured atheromatous
  Hollenhorst
  intraluminal
  obstructive
  sessile
  stenotic
  ulcerated
plaque cracker, LeVeen
Plasbumin
Plasma TFE vascular graft
plasma thromboplastin component (PTC)
plasma viscosity
plasma volume expander (Hespan or hetastarch)
Plasmalyte A cardioplegic solution
Plasmalyte (solution in liver transplant procedures)
Plasmanate
plasmapheresis
Plasmatein
plasma, fresh frozen
Plasma-Plex
plasmin
platelet, HLA-type specific
platelet adhesiveness
platelet aggregation
platelet count
pledget
  cotton
  oval
  Teflon
  Teflon felt
pledgeted Ethibond suture
Plegisol cardioplegic solution

Plesch test
plethora
plethysmograph, Medsonic
plethysmography
   impedance (IPG)
   strain-gauge
   venous
Pleur-evac suction tube
pleura
   mediastinal
   parietal
   pericardiac
   visceral
pleural adhesion
pleural space
pleuritic pain
pleurodesis
pleuropericardial incision
plexogenic pulmonary arteriopathy (PPA)
plication, annular
plication repair of flail leaflet
plop, tumor
PLR (peripheral laser recanalization)
PLT (primed lymphocyte test)
plug
   Alcock catheter
   Teflon Bardic
PM (posterior mitral)
PMD (papillary muscle dysfunction)
PMI (point of maximal impulse; maximum intensity)
PML (posterior mitral leaflet)
PMT AccuSpan tissue expander
PMV (percutaneous mitral balloon valvotomy; valvuloplasty)
PMV (prolapsed mitral valve)
PNC (premature nodal contraction)
PND (paroxysmal nocturnal dyspnea)
pneumopericardium
pneuPAC ventilator/resuscitator
PNH (paroxysmal nocturnal hemoglobinuria)
pO_2

pocket
   pacemaker tissue
   subcutaneous pacemaker
point
   A
   C
   D
   de Mussy
   E
   Erb
   F
   J
   Mussy
   null
   O
point of Arrhigi
point of maximal intensity (PMI)
point of maximum impulse (PMI)
polarcardiography
polarity
polarizing
Polhemus-Schafer-Ivemark syndrome
polyarteritis nodosa
polycythemia
Polydek suture
PolyFlex lead pacemaker
polygelin colloid contrast medium
polymorphic ventricular tachycardia
Polystan perfusion cannula
Polystan venous return catheter
polyurethane foam embolus
pooling of blood in extremities
pop-off suture
popliteal pulse
popliteal space
Poppen-Blalock carotid clamp
poppet
   ball
   barium-impregnated
   disk
   prosthetic valve
porcine heterograft
porcine xenograft bioprosthesis

port
  injection
  Quinton vascular access
  side-arm pressure
  vent
portal hypertension
Portnoy ventricular cannula
position
  anterior oblique
  Fowler
  left anterior oblique (LAO)
  left lateral decubitus
  pulmonary capillary wedge
  right anterior oblique (RAO)
  squatting
  steep Trendelenburg
  wedge
positive deflection on EKG
Positrol II catheter
positron emission tomography (PET)
positron emitters
postangioplasty stenosis
postcardiotomy intra-aortic balloon pumping
postcardiotomy syndrome
postcommissurotomy syndrome
postconversion electrocardiogram
postmyocardiotomy infarction
postpericardiotomy syndrome
poststreptococcal inflammatory process
posterior descending artery (PDA)
posterior inferior communicating artery (PICA)
posterior table
posterolateral
posterolateral branch
posteroseptal Kent bundle
postexercise tracing
postinfarction ventriculoseptal defect
postinfarction course
postmyocardial infarction syndrome
postoperative pericarditis
postpericardiotomy syndrome
postphlebitic syndrome
poststenotic dilatation
postural
Potain sign
potassium chloride cardioplegia
potassium-sparing effect
potential
  action
  membrane
  resting membrane
  ventricular late (VLP)
Potts anastomosis
Potts aortic clamp
Potts bronchus forceps
Potts bulldog forceps
Potts clamp
Potts coarctation clamp
Potts needle
Potts patent ductus clamp
Potts scissors
Potts 60° angled scissors
Potts shunt
Potts thumb forceps
Potts vascular forceps
Potts vascular scissors
Potts-Niedner clamp
Potts-Satinsky clamp
Potts-Smith aortic occlusion clamp
Potts-Smith scissors
Potts-Smith side-to-side anastomosis
Potts-Smith tissue forceps
Potts-Smith vascular scissors
pouch, pacemaker generator
pounding, heart
power pack, abdominal
PP interval
PPA (plexogenic pulmonary arteriopathy)
PPAS (peripheral pulmonary artery stenosis)
PPH (primary pulmonary hypertension)
PPM (posterior papillary muscle)
P:QRS ratio

PR interval
  prolongation of
  shortening of
PR segment, depressed
PRA (plasma renin activity) test
preangioplasty stenosis
precatheterization
preclot the graft
preclotting of graft
precordial honk
precordial lead
precordial motion
precordial palpation
precordial thump
precordium
  active
  anterior
  bulging of
preductal coarctation of aorta
pre-ejection period (PEP)
preexcitation, ventricular
preexcitation syndrome
pre-exercise resting supine EKG
preinfarction syndrome
preload, cardiac
premature atrial complex or contraction (PAC)
premature mid-diastolic closure of mitral valve
premature valve closure
premature ventricular complex or contraction (PVC)
preoperative resting MUGA scan
preperitoneal fat
prescription (Rx)
pressor therapy
pressure
  "a" wave (left or right atrial catheterization)
  ambulant venous (AVP)
  ankle-arm
  AO (aorta)
  aortic
  arterial (ART)
  atmospheres of

pressure *(cont.)*
  blood (BP)
  brachial artery end-diastolic
  brachial artery peak systolic
  c wave (right atrial catheterization)
  capillary
  central aortic
  central venous (CVP)
  chest
  continuous positive airway (CPAP)
  coronary wedge
  critical closing (CCP)
  cuff blood
  diastolic
  diastolic blood (DBP)
  diastolic filling (DFP)
  diastolic pulmonary artery
  distal coronary perfusion
  Doppler blood
  end-diastolic (right ventricular catheterization)
  endocardial
  end-systolic (ESP)
  femoral artery (FAP)
  filling
  high blood (HBP)
  intracardiac
  intraventricular
  in vivo balloon
  jugular venous
  LA (left atrium)
  left atrial (LAP)
  left-sided heart
  left subclavian central venous (LSCVP)
  left ventricular (LV)
  left ventricular end-diastolic (LVEDP)
  left ventricular filling
  left ventricular peak systolic
  left ventricular systolic (LVS)
  manual
  maximum inflation

pressure *(cont.)*
  mean
  mean aortic
  mean arterial (MAP)
  mean blood
  mean brachial artery
  mean left atrial
  mean pulmonary artery (MPAP)
  mean pulmonary artery wedge
  mean right atrial
  PA (pulmonary artery) systolic
  PAD (pulmonary artery diastolic)
  PAS (pulmonary artery systolic)
  peak systolic aortic (PSAP)
  peak systolic (right ventricular catheterization)
  phasic
  positive end-expiratory (PEEP)
  pulmonary artery (PAP)
  pulmonary artery diastolic (PAD)
  pulmonary artery end-diastolic (PAEDP)
  pulmonary artery mean (PAM)
  pulmonary artery peak systolic
  pulmonary artery systolic (PAS)
  pulmonary artery wedge (PAWP)
  pulmonary artery/pulmonary capillary wedge
  pulmonary capillary (PCP)
  pulmonary capillary wedge (PCWP)
  pulmonary venous capillary (PVC)
  pulse
  PV (pulmonary vein)
  PVC (pulmonary venous capillary)
  RA (right atrial)
  right atrial (RAP)
  right heart
  right subclavian central venous (RSCVP)
  right ventricular (RVP)

pressure *(cont.)*
  right ventricular diastolic (RVD)
  right ventricular end-diastolic
  right ventricular peak systolic
  right ventricular systolic (RVS)
  right ventricular volume
  right-sided heart
  RV (right ventricular)
  RVD (right ventricular diastolic)
  RVS (right ventricular systolic)
  stump
  supersystemic pulmonary artery
  SVC (superior vena cava)
  systemic
  systolic
  systolic blood (SBP)
  torr
  transcutaneous oxygen
  v wave (left or right atrial catheterization)
  venous
  wedge
  withdrawal
  x' wave (right atrial cath)
  y wave (right atrial cath)
  z point (left or right atrial cath)
pressure injector
pressure measurement
pressure readings
pressure sensation
pressure transducer
pressure waveform
pressure-like sensation in chest
presyncopal episode
presyncope
presystolic murmur (PSM)
presystolic pulsation
pretibial edema
Price-Thomas bronchial forceps
Prima pacemaker
principle
  Doppler
  Fick
  Frank-Starling
  indicator fractionation

Prinzmetal variant angina
Prism-CL pacemaker
prism method for ventricular volume
proarrhythmia
prob (probable, probably)
probe
　blood flow
　cardiac
　Chandler V-pacing
　Doppler flow
　echocardiographic
　electromagnetic flow
　Hagar
　hand-held exploring electrode
　nuclear
　Parsonnet
　Siemens-Elema AB pulse transducer
　Teflon
　temperature
　transesophageal
Probe balloon-on-a-wire dilatation system, USCI
probe-patent foramen ovale
probing catheter, USCI
procedure (see *operation*)
process
　left ventricular posterior superior
　xiphoid
proconvertin blood coagulation factor
prodromal symptoms
profile
　automated physiologic
　biophysical (BPP)
　serum lipid
Profile Plus dilatation catheter, USCI
Proflex 5 dilatation catheter
profunda Dacron patchplasty
profunda femoris artery
profundaplasty
Programalith pacemaker
programmability of pacemaker rate

programmed electrical stimulation (PES)
Programmer III
programming
　bidirectional pacemaker
　phantom pacemaker
　unidirectional pacemaker
progression, poor R wave (PRWP)
progressive care unit
projection (see also *view*)
　anterior
　left anterior oblique (LAO)
　left lateral
　right anterior oblique (RAO)
　65° LAO
　steep left anterior oblique
　30° LAO
prolapse
　mitral
　mitral valve (MVP)
　tricuspid valve
prolapsed mitral valve leaflets
Prolene suture
proliferation, intimal
Prolith pacemaker
prolongation of QRS interval
prolongation of QT wave
prophylactic implantation of pacemaker
prophylactic penicillin
prophylaxis
　endocarditis
　SBE (subacute bacterial endocarditis)
prostacycline
prostaglandin E_1
prosthesis (see also *valve*)
　aortic valve
　aortofemoral
　ball-and-cage valve
　ball-cage
　ball valve
　Beall disk valve
　Beall mitral valve
　bifurcated aortofemoral

prosthesis *(cont.)*
  bi-leaflet valve
  Bionit vascular
  bioprosthesis
  Bjork-Shiley aortic valve
  Bjork-Shiley convexo-concave
    60° valve
  Bjork-Shiley mitral valve
  Bjork-Shiley monostrut 72° valve
  Bjork-Shiley valve
  bovine pericardial
  Braunwald-Cutter ball valve
  caged ball valve
  Carpentier annuloplasty ring
  Carpentier-Edwards valve
  convexo-concave valve
  Cross-Jones disk valve
  Cutter aortic valve
  Cutter-Smeloff cardiac valve
  DeBakey ball valve
  De Vega
  Delrin frame of valve
  disk valve
  femorofemoral crossover
  golf tee-shaped polyvinyl
  Hall-Kaster mitral valve
  Hall-Kaster tilting-disk valve
  Hancock aortic valve
  Hancock mitral valve
  Hancock porcine valve
  Ionescu-Shiley aortic valve
  Kastec mitral valve
  Kay-Shiley disk valve
  Lillehei valve
  Lillehei-Cruz-Kaster
  Lillehei-Kaster mitral valve
  Lo-Por vascular graft
  Magovern ball valve
  Magovern-Cromie
  Meadox woven velour
  Medtronic-Hall tilting-disk valve
  Microknit vascular graft
  Milliknit vascular graft
  monostrut valve
  Omniscience tilting-disk valve

prosthesis *(cont.)*
  polyvinyl
  porcine heterograft
  Smeloff-Cutter ball valve
  St. Jude Medical aortic valve
  St. Jude Medical bi-leaflet
    tilting-disk aortic valve
  St. Jude valve
  Starr-Edwards aortic valve
  Starr-Edwards ball valve
  Starr-Edwards disk valve
  Sutter-Smeloff heart valve
  tilting-disk aortic valve
  USCI Sauvage EXS side-limb
protection
  cardiac
  myocardial
protein, total
Protenate
prothrombin time (PT)
pro time (prothrombin time)
protocol
  advanced cardiac life support
    (ACLS)
  Balke treadmill stress test
  Balke-Ware treadmill exercise
  Bruce treadmill exercise stress
  cardiac rehabilitation
  CCU
  Ellestad treadmill exercise
  exercise
  Kattus treadmill exercise
  Mayo exercise treadmill
  McHenry treadmill exercise
  modified Balke treadmill exercise
  modified Bruce treadmill exercise
  modified treadmill
  Naughton treadmill exercise
  Naughton-Balke treadmill
  pacing
  Reeves treadmill exercise
  rule out MI (ROMI)
  Sheffield exercise test
  Sheffield modification of Bruce
    treadmill

protocol *(cont.)*
    Sheffield treadmill exercise
    slow USAFSAM treadmill exercise
    soft rule out MI
    standard Bruce treadmill exercise
    Stanford treadmill exercise
    TIMI II (thrombolysis in myocardial infarction)
    USAFSAM treadmill exercise
protodiastolic reversal of blood flow
proximal circumflex artery
proximal coronary sinus (CS)
proximal and distal portion of vessel
proximal segment
PR segment depression
Pruitt-Inahara carotid shunt
pruned appearance of pulmonary vasculature
PRWP (poor R wave progression)
PS (pulmonic stenosis)
P/S flow ratio (pulmonic/systemic)
PSA (pacing system analyzer)
PSAP (peak systolic aortic pressure)
pseudoaneurysm
pseudoclaudication syndrome
pseudohemophilia, hereditary
pseudoincisura
pseudoinfarction
pseudolupus secondary to procainamide
pseudotruncus arteriosus
pseudoxanthoma elasticum
PSG (peak systolic gradient)
psi ("sigh") (pounds per square inch)
PSM (presystolic murmur)
PSVT (paroxysmal supraventricular tachycardia)
PSVT, slow-fast intranodal
psychosis, postcardiotomy
PT (prothrombin time), prolonged
PT/PTT (prothrombin time/partial thromboplastin time)
PTA (percutaneous transluminal angioplasty)
PTBD (percutaneous transluminal balloon dilatation)
PTC (plasma thromboplastin component)
PTCA (percutaneous transluminal coronary angioplasty)
PTCA catheter; catheterization
PTCA coronary angiogram
PTFE (polytetrafluoroethylene) graft
PTFE arterial graft material
PTL (posterior tricuspid leaflet)
PTMC (percutaneous transvenous mitral commissurotomy)
PTT (partial thromboplastin time; pulmonary transit time)
Puig Massana-Shiley annuloplasty valve
pullback, left heart
pullback across the aortic valve
pullback arterial markings
pullback from ventricle
pulmonary arterial input impedance
pulmonary arterial markings
pulmonary arterial vent
pulmonary artery end-diastolic pressure (PAEDP)
pulmonary AV O_2 difference
pulmonary bed
pulmonary capillary wedge pressure (PCWP)
pulmonary congestion
pulmonary flotation catheter
pulmonary hypertension
pulmonary outflow tract
pulmonary/systemic flow ratio
pulmonary toilet
pulmonary vascular markings; pattern
pulmonary vascular resistance (PVR)
pulmonary venous congestion
pulmonary wedge pressure (PWP)

pulmonic valve stenosis
Pulsar NI pacemaker
pulsatile abdominal mass
pulsatile assist device (PAD)
pulsatile perfusion
pulsation
  capillary
  carotid arterial
  expansile
  hepatic vein
  jugular venous
  precordial
  presystolic
  suprasternal
pulse
  "a" peak of jugular venous
  abdominal
  absence of
  absent
  allorhythmic
  alternating
  anacrotic
  anadicrotic
  anatricotic
  apex
  apical
  arterial
  biferious
  bifid arterial
  bigeminal
  bilaterally symmetric
  bisferious
  bounding
  brachial
  C point of cardiac apex
  c wave of jugular venous
  cannon ball
  capillary
  cardiac apex
  carotid
  carotid arterial (CAR)
  catadicrotic
  character of
  collapsing
  Corrigan

pulse *(cont.)*
  coupled
  delayed femoral
  dicrotic
  dicrotic arterial
  distal
  Doppler
  dorsal pedis
  dorsalis pedis
  dropped-beat
  external carotid
  femoral
  filiform
  formicant
  full
  h peak of jugular venous
  hard
  high-tension
  incisura of
  intermittent
  irregular
  irregularly irregular
  jerky
  jugular
  jugular venous
  Kussmaul paradoxical
  labile
  lower extremity
  low-tension
  Monneret
  movable
  nonpalpable
  palpable
  paradoxic
  paradoxical
  parvus
  peripheral
  pistol-shot
  plateau-type
  polycrotic
  popliteal
  posterior tibial
  pressure
  quadrigeminal
  quick

pulse *(cont.)*
  Quincke
  radial
  rapid
  regular
  regularly irregular
  retrosternal
  Riegel
  running
  slow
  spike-and-dome
  strong
  symmetric
  tardus
  thready
  tidal wave
  tremulous
  tricrotic
  trigeminal
  trip-hammer
  ulnar
  undulating
  v peak of jugular venous
  vermicular
  water-hammer
  wiry
  x depression of jugular venous
  x descent of jugular venous
  y descent of jugular venous
pulse amplitude
pulse character
pulse deficit
pulse generator of pacemaker (see *generator*)
pulse pressure
pulse rate, baseline standing
pulse wave
pulseless bradycardia; disease
pulselessness
pulses, unequal
pulsus alternans
pulsus bisferiens
pulsus paradoxus
pulsus parvus et tardus
pulsus tardus

pump
  angle port
  blood
  calcium
  cardiac balloon
  Cormed
  Datascope System 90 balloon
  intra-aortic balloon (IABP)
  ion
  Novacore
  priming of the
  pulmonary artery balloon (PABP)
  sodium
  sump
  Thoratec
  Travenol infusion
  volumetric infusion
pump failure, Cedars-Sinai classification of
pump oxygenator
pump perfusionist
pump technician
pumping, postcardiotomy intra-aortic balloon
pumping capacity of heart
punch
  aortic
  circular
  Goosen vascular
  Hancock aortic
  Karp aortic
  Medtronic aortic
  Sweet sternal
puncture
  arterial
  groin
  percutaneous
  venous
  ventricular
Purkinje cells; fibers
Purkinje network
Purmann method
purpura, thrombotic thrombocytopenic

PV (pulmonic valve)
PVB (premature ventricular beat)
PVC (premature ventricular contraction)
   bigeminal
   early-cycle
   multifocal
   multiform
   paired
   unifocal
PVCs (preventricular contractions)
PVCs in a bigeminal pattern
PVD (peripheral vascular disease)
PVER (paced ventricular evoked response)
PVOD (pulmonary veno-occlusive disease)
PVR (peripheral vascular resistance; pulmonary vascular resistance; pulse volume recorder)
PW (posterior wall)
PWT (posterior wall thickness)
PYP (pyrophosphate) scan
pyramid method for ventricular volume
pyridoxilated stroma-free hemoglobin (SFHb)
pyrophosphate (PYP) scan
pyrosis (heartburn)

Q

Q wave
   nondiagnostic
   pathologic
   septal
Q-cath catheterization recording system
QH interval of jugular venous pulse
QOL (quality of life) index
QO_2 (oxygen consumption)
Q Port
QR pattern
QRS complex (see also *complex*)
   fusion
   normal voltage
   preexcited
   slurring of
   wide
QRS complex duration
QRS duration
QRS interval
QRS loop
QRS score
QRS vector
QRS-T angle, wide
QRS-T complex
QS deflection
QS wave
QS_1 interval
QS_2 interval
Q-Stress treadmill
QT interval
QT syndrome
QT_c interval (corrected QT interval)
QU interval
quadrigeminy
quadripolar catheter
Quain fatty heart
quality of life (QOL) index
Quanticor catheter
quantitation of ischemic muscle
Quantum pacemaker
Quénu-Muret sign
Quick test
Quik-Prep, Quinton
Quincke disease
Quincke pulse
Quincke sign
Quinton catheter
Quinton computerized exercise EKG system
Quinton electrode
Quinton Quik-Prep
Quinton vascular access port

R

R and S wave pattern over precordium, reversal of
R wave
  low-amplitude
  tall
  upright
R wave of jugular venous pulse
R wave upstroke, slurred
R wave progression, poor
R' (R prime) wave
R-2 pad
R-lactate enzymatic monotest
R/O (rule out)
RS4 pacemaker
R/S ratio; wave ratio
R-on-T phenomenon
R-on-T ventricular premature contraction
R-to-R scanning
RA (right atrial) pressure
Raaf Cath (vascular catheter)
RAAPI (resting ankle-arm pressure index)
RACAT (rapid acquisition computed axial tomography)
racing of heart
RAD (right axis deviation)
radial artery catheter
radial pulse
radioimmunoassay
radioisotope
  carbon-11 palmitic acid radioactive
  indium-111
  iodine-123 (heptadecanoic acid)
  iodine-123 (pentylpentadecanoic acid (IPPA)
  iodine-125
  iodine-131
  rubidium-82
  technetium-99m

radioisotope *(cont.)*
  thallium-201
radionuclide, gold-195m
radionuclide angiocardiography
radionuclide angiogram (RNA)
radiotracer
RAE (right atrial enlargement)
rake retractor
rale, rales
  basilar
  bibasilar
  crackling
  crepitant
  dry
  moist
  sibilant
  sonorous
  wet
ramus branch
ramus intermedius artery
ramus medianus
Randall stone forceps for thromboendarterectomy
RAO (right anterior oblique)
RAO position for cardiac catheterization
RAO view on cardiac catheterization
RAP (right atrial pressure)
raphe
rapid atrial pacing
Rashkind atrial septostomy
Rashkind balloon atrial septostomy
Rashkind blade septostomy
Rashkind septostomy balloon catheter
Rashkind-Miller atrial septostomy
rasp, raspatory
  Alexander-Faraheuf rib
  Doyen rib
Rastelli operation; repair

rate
  atrial (AR)
  auricular
  basic
  echo intensity disappearance
  erythrocyte sedimentation (ESR)
  exercise-induced heart
  heart (HR)
  KVO (keep vein open)
  left ventricular filling
  maximal heart
  maximum predicted heart (MPHR)
  peak exercise heart
  peak filling (PFR)
  percent of predicted
  predetermined heart
  predicted maximum heart
  pulse
  resting heart
  respiratory
  sed (sedimentation)
  sinus
  slew (SR)
  stroke ejection
  systolic ejection (SER)
  target heart
  time-to-peak filling (TPFR)
  ventricular
  washout
  Westergren sedimentation
rate and incline of treadmill
rate and rhythm of heartbeat
rate and rhythm, regular (RRR)
rate hysteresis
rate-responsive pacemaker, permanent
RATG (rabbit antithymocyte globulin)
ratio
  AH:HA
  AO/AC (aortic valve opening/aortic valve closing)
  aortic root
  cardiothoracic (CTR)

ratio *(cont.)*
  CK/AST
  conduction (number of P waves to number of QRS)
  E/A (on echocardiography)
  ESP/ESV
  ESWI/ESVI (end-systolic wall stress index/end-systolic volume)
  left ventricular systolic time interval
  mean total cholesterol/HDL
  PASP/SASP (pulmonary to systemic arterial systolic pressure)
  P:QRS
  P/S flow (pulmonic/systemic)
  pulmonary to systemic flow
  pulmonary/systemic flow
  R/S amplitude
  R/S wave
  $RV_6:RV_5$ voltage
  RVP/LVP (right ventricular to left ventricular systolic pressure)
  septal to free wall
  T/D (thickness to diameter of ventricle)
  VLDL-TG/HDL-C
rauwolfia derivative
Raynaud disease; syndrome
Raynaud phenomenon
Ray-Tec x-ray detectable sponge
RBBB (right bundle branch block)
RBC (red blood cell) count
RBC indices
  MCH (mean corpuscular hemoglobin)
  MCHC (mean corpuscular hemoglobin concentration)
  MCV (mean corpuscular volume)
RBC, technetium-99m labeled
RCA (right coronary artery)
RCM (restricted cardiomyopathy)
reabsorbable suture

reaction recovery time
Real coronary artery scissors
real-time ultrasonography
ream out (verb)
recalcitrant
recanalization
   argon laser
   percutaneous transluminal
      coronary
   peripheral laser (PLR)
recanalized artery
receptor
   adrenergic
   alpha
   alpha-adrenergic
   alpha$_1$-adrenergic
   beta
   beta-adrenergic
   beta$_1$-adrenergic
   beta$_2$-adrenergic
   LDL
recessed balloon septostomy
   catheter
reciprocal changes
recoarctation
recoil, catheter
recombinant tissue-type plasminogen activator (rtPA)
reconstitution via a profunda
reconstitution via collaterals
reconstruction
   aortic
   patch graft
   transannular patch
recovery period of myocardium
recurrent intractable ventricular
   tachycardia
recurring ectopic beats
red cell aplasia
Redifocus guide wire
RediFurl TaperSeal IAB catheter
redirection of inferior vena cava
redistributed thallium scan
redistribution myocardial image

redistribution of pulmonary
   vascular blood flow
Reed ventriculorrhaphy
reedswitch of pacemaker
reentrant circuit
reentrant loop
reentry
   atrial
   AV nodal
   Bachmann bundle
   bundle branch (BBR)
   intra-atrial
   SA nodal
   sinus nodal
Reeves treadmill exercise protocol
REFI (regional ejection fraction
   image)
reflection, epicardial
reflex
   abdominocardiac
   Abrams heart
   Aschner
   atriopressor
   Bainbridge
   baroreceptor
   Bezold-Jarisch
   bregmocardiac
   carotid sinus
   coronary
   Cushing
   deep tendon (DTR)
   Erben
   hyperactive carotid sinus
   hepatojugular
   Livierato
   Lovén
   oculocardiac
   psychocardiac
   pulmonocoronary
   vascular
   vasopressor
   viscerocardiac
reflux, hepatojugular
refractoriness, ventricular

refractory congestive heart failure
refractory period (see *period*)
refractory to medical therapy
Reg. (regurgitation)
regimen, stepped-care antihypertensive
regional ejection fraction image
  (REFI)
regional left ventricular function
regional myocardial uptake of
  thallium
regional wall motion abnormality
regular rate and rhythm
regurgitant flow
regurgitant jet
regurgitant mitral valve murmur
regurgitant velocity
regurgitation (Reg.)
  aortic (AR)
  congenital mitral (CMR)
  Dexter-Grossman classification
    of mitral
  Grossman scale for
  ischemically mediated mitral
  mitral (MR)
  mitral valve
  paravalvular
  pulmonary
  pulmonic
  pulmonic valve
  tricuspid (TR)
  tricuspid valve
  trivial mitral
  valvular
rehabilitation, cardiac
rehabilitation exercises
Rehbein rib spreader
Rehfuss tube
rehydrated
reinfarction
Reinhoff clamp
Reinhoff-Finochietto rib spreader
relative refractory period (RRP)
relaxation, isovolumelic (IVR)
renin-angiotensin system

Renografin contrast medium
Renografin-76/50% saline solution,
  hand-agitated
Renovist contrast medium
Renovist II contrast medium
Rentrop infusion catheter
reperfuse, reperfusion
reperfusion injury
replacement
  aortic valve (AVR)
  mitral valve (MVR)
repolarization
  atrial
  early
  ventricular
resectability
resection (see also *operation*)
  endocardial-to-epicardial
  infundibular
  selective subendocardial
  transmural
  wedge-shaped sleeve aneurysm
reserve
  coronary flow (CFR)
  left ventricular systolic func-
    tional
  myocardial perfusion (MPR)
  regional contractile
  stenotic flow (SFR)
  ventricular
residual gradient
resistance
  airway
  arteriolar
  calculated
  coronary
  peripheral
  peripheral vascular (PVR)
  pulmonary
  pulmonary arteriolar
  pulmonary vascular (PVR)
  systemic
  systemic vascular (SVR)
  total peripheral (TPR)
  total pulmonary (TPR)

resistance *(cont.)*
  vascular
    Wood units index of
respirations
  labored
  unlabored
respirator (see *ventilator*)
response
  abnormal ejection fraction
  rapid ventricular
  slow ventricular
rest LV function
rest RV function
rest thallium-201 myocardial
  imaging
restenosis
resting electrocardiogram
resting end-systolic wall stress
resting heart rate
resting MUGA scan, preoperative
resuscitation
  cardiopulmonary (CPR)
  closed chest cardiopulmonary
  mouth-to-mouth
reticulocyte count
retinal exudate
retinopathy, hypertensive
retraction, postrheumatic cusp
retractions
  intercostal
  substernal
  suprasternal
retractor
  Allison lung
  Ankeney sternal
  Army-Navy
  atrial
  Beckman
  Burford
  Cooley atrial
  Crawford aortic
  Cushing vein
  Davidson
  Davidson scapular
  Deaver

retractor *(cont.)*
  DeBakey-Cooley
  Favaloro sternal
  Finochietto
  Garrett
  Gelpi
  Haight-Finochietto rib
  Harrington
  Hartzler rib
  Himmelstein sternal
  Kelly
  Kirklin atrial
  leaflet
  lung
  malleable
  Miller-Senn
  Ochsner
  rake
  Richardson
  Sachs vein
  Sauerbruch
  self-retaining
  Semb lung
  Senn
  sternal
  U.S. Army
  vein
  Volkmann
  Weitlaner
retrograde aortogram
retrograde atherectomy
retrograde atrial activation mapping
retrograde blood flow across valve
retrograde conduction
retrograde fashion
  advanced in a
  catheter advanced in a
retrograde filling
retrograde injection
retrograde percutaneous femoral artery approach for cardiac cath
retrograde refractory period
retroperfusion, synchronized
retroperitoneal hematoma
retrosternal chest pain

revascularization
  coronary
  myocardial
  surgical
revascularized
reversed arm leads
reversed coarctation
rewarm, rewarmed, rewarming
Reynolds number
Reynolds vascular clamp
RF (radiofrequency; rapid filling; rheumatic fever)
RF (radiofrequency-generated thermal) balloon catheter
RF wave of cardiac apex pulse
RFP (rapid filling period)
RFW (rapid filling wave)
rhabdomyoma, cardiac
RHD (rheumatic heart disease)
Rheomacrodex
rheumatic fever (RF)
rheumatic heart disease (RHD)
rheumatoid arthritis (RA) factor
rhonchus, rhonchi
RHV (right ventricular hypertrophy)
rhythm
  accelerated idioventricular
  AV (atrioventricular)
  AV junctional
  AV nodal (AVNR)
  baseline
  bigeminal
  cardiac
  coronary sinus (CSR)
  coupled
  ectopic
  embryocardia
  escape
  fibrillation
  gallop
  idioventricular
  irregularly irregular heart
  junctional escape
  mu
  nodal

rhythm *(cont.)*
  nodal escape
  normal sinus (NSR)
  paced
  pacemaker
  parasystolic
  pendulum
  predominant
  pulseless idioventricular
  reciprocal
  regular sinus (RSR)
  regularly irregular heart
  sinus
  slow escape
  systolic
  tic-tac
  ventricular
  wide complex
rhythm disturbance
rhythm strip
rib guillotine
Richardson retractor
ridge, supra-aortic
Riegel pulse
right and retrograde left heart catheterization
right-angle chest tube
right ankle indices
right anterior oblique (RAO) position
right atrial enlargement
right axis deviation
right bundle branch block with left anterior (or posterior) hemiblock
right internal jugular artery
right-sided heart failure
right upper sternal border
right ventricular assist device (RVAD)
right ventricular conduction defect
right ventricular hypertrophy
right ventricular lift
right ventricular myocardial aplasia
right ventricular outflow tract
right ventricular systolic time interval

right-to-left shunt with pulmonic stenosis
RIND (reversible intermittent or ischemic neurologic deficit)
Rindfleisch, fold of
ring
  atrioventricular
  Carpentier
  Crawford suture
  double-flanged valve sewing
  Duran annuloplasty
  mitral valve
  prosthetic valve sewing
  prosthetic valve suture
  supra-annular suture
  tricuspid valve
  universal valve prosthesis sewing
  valve
risk, surgical
risk factors for cardiac disease
  age
  alcohol consumption
  alcoholism
  blood pressure
  caffeine consumption
  cigarette smoking
  coffee drinker
  coronary disease
  diabetes mellitus, type I
  diabetes mellitus, type II
  diet
  elevated blood lipids
  environment
  familial disposition
  gender (male more than female)
  genetic
  heredity
  high blood pressure (HBP)
  high plasma LDL
  hypercholesterolemia
  hyperlipidemia
  hypertension
  hypertriglyceridemia
  lack of exercise
  low plasma HDL

risk factors *(cont.)*
  obesity
  oral contraceptive use
  personality type A
  physical inactivity
  race
  saturated fat consumption
  sedentary lifestyle
  sex (gender; male more than female)
  smoking
  stress
  tobacco use
  type A personality
Riva-Rocci manometer
Rivero-Carvallo maneuver; sign
RMVT (repetitive monomorphic ventricular tachycardia)
RNA (radionuclide angiogram), gated
RNV (radionuclide ventriculogram)
Rochester-Mixter artery forceps
Rodriguez catheter
roentgenkymography
roentgenogram, chest
Roger disease
Roger murmur
Rokitansky disease
Romano-Ward syndrome
Romhilt-Estes score for left ventricular hypertrophy
ROMI (rule out myocardial infarction); also ROMIed (verb)
rongeur
  Bethune
  Cushing
  Giertz
  Sauerbruch
  Semb
root, aortic
Rosen guide wire
Rosenbach syndrome
Rotablator atherectomy device
Rotch sign
Rotex II biopsy needle

Roth spot
Rougnon-Heberden disease
Royal Flush angiographic flush catheter
Rozanski precordial lead placement system
RP interval
RPA (right pulmonary artery)
RPV (right pulmonary vein)
RR cycle
RR interval
RRP (rate-responsive pacing; relative refractory period)
RR' (RR prime) pattern
RRR (regular rate and rhythm)
RS complex
rS deflection
RS4 pacemaker
RSCVP (right subclavian central venous pressure)
RSR (regular sinus rhythm)
RSR' triphasic pattern (on EKG)
RSV (regurgitant stroke volume)
rtPA (recombinant tissue-type plasminogen activator)
rub, pericardial friction
rubber band, Vesseloops
Rubinstein-Taybi syndrome
rubidium-82 imaging
Ruel forceps
rule, Simpson
rule of bigeminy
rule out (R/O)
rule out myocardial infarction (ROMI)
rumble
   Austin Flint
   booming
   diastolic
   mid-diastolic (or middiastolic)
   protodiastolic
Rumel catheter
Rumel myocardial clamp; tourniquet
Rumel thoracic forceps

runoff
   aortic
   arterial
   digital
   distal
runoff arteriogram
runs of arrhythmia
runs of PVCs
runs of tachycardia
runs of ventricular tachycardia, spontaneously occurring
rupture
   abdominal aortic aneurysm
   cardiac
   interventricular septal
   papillary muscle
   ventricular free wall
   ventricular septal
Russian tissue forceps
RV (right ventricle) pressure
RV strain
$RV_6:RV_5$ voltage ratio
RVA (right ventricular apical) electrogram
RVAD (right ventricular assist device), Thoratec
RVBF (reversed vertebral blood flow)
RVCD (right ventricular conduction defect)
RVD (right ventricular diastolic) pressure
RVD (right ventricular dimension)
RVE (right ventricular enlargement)
RVEDP (right ventricular end-diastolic pressure)
RVEF (right ventricular ejection fraction)
RVFW (right ventricular free wall)
RVH (right ventricular hypertrophy)
RVID (right ventricular internal diameter)
RVM (right ventricular mass)
RVOT (right ventricular outflow tract)

RVP (right ventricular pressure)
RVP/LVP (right ventricular to left ventricular systolic pressure) ratio
RVS (right ventricular systolic) pressure
RVSTI (right ventricular systolic time interval)
RVSW (right ventricular stroke work)
Rx (prescription)

S

S wave
  deep
  slurred
  wide
S_1 (first heart sound)
S_2 (second heart sound)
  fixed splitting of
  paradoxical splitting of
  physiologically split
S_3 (third heart sound)
S_4 (fourth heart sound)
S_3 gallop
S_2OS inteval
S_1Q_3 pattern
$S_1Q_3T_3$ pattern
S_1S_2 interval
S_1S_3 interval
$S_1S_2S_3$ pattern
SaO_2 (arterial oxygen saturation)
SA (sinoatrial) node
SA nodal reentry tachycardia
SAB (sinoatrial block)
sac, pericardial
Sachs vein retractor
SACT (sinoatrial conduction time)
saddle embolus
Sade modification of Norwood procedure
SAECG (signal-averaged electrocardiogram)
sagging ST segment
Salibi carotid artery clamp

saline
  cold
  half normal (0.45% NaCl)
  heparinized
  iced
  normal (0.9% NaCl)
  topical cold
saline loading
saline solution
Salkowski test
salt restriction; restricted diet
salvage of limb
salvage of myocardium
salvo of ventricular tachycardia
salvos of premature ventricular complexes
SAM (systolic anterior motion; systolic aortic motion)
Samuels forceps
Samuels hemoclip
SAN (sinoatrial node)
Sanchez-Cascos cardioauditory syndrome
sandbag
sandwich patch closure, anterior
Sansom sign
saphenofemoral junction
saphenous vein graft
saphenous vein, greater
sarcoma
  cardiac
  Kaposi epicardial

Sarns aortic arch cannula
Sarns electric saw
Sarns two-stage cannula
Sarot artery forceps
Sarot bronchus clamp
Satinsky aortic clamp
Satinsky scissors
Satinsky vascular clamp
Satinsky vena cava clamp
saturation
　arterial oxygen
　mixed venous
　oxygen (O$_2$)
Sauerbruch retractor
Sauerbruch rib shears
Sauerbruch rongeur
Sauvage filamentous velour Dacron arterial graft material
saw
　Gigli
　Hall sternal
　oscillating sternotomy
　Sarns electric
　sternotomy
　Stryker
SB (sinus bradycardia)
SBE (subacute bacterial endocarditis) prophylaxis
SBF (systemic blood flow)
SBP (systolic blood pressure)
scalar EKG
scalenus anticus syndrome
scalloped commissure
scalloping
scalpel
scan, scanning
　cine CT
　dipyridamole thallium-201
　duplex
　gated equilibrium blood pool
　isotope-labeled fibrinogen leg
　MUGA (multiple gated acquisition) blood pool radionuclide
　perfusion lung
　PET

scan *(cont.)*
　redistributed thallium
　rest thallium-201
　resting MUGA
　R-to-R
　SPECT thallium
　stress thallium
　technetium-99m pyrophosphate myocardial
　ultrafast CT
　ventilation-perfusion
scanography
scar
　infarcted
　myocardial
　nonviable
　well-demarcated
　zipper
scar formation on myocardium
Scarpa method
Schede thoracoplasty
Scheie syndrome
Schellong-Strisower phenomenon
Schiff test
Schneider catheter
Schneider PTCA instruments
Schneider-Shiley catheter
Schnidt clamp; passer
Schonander film changer; technique
Schoonmaker femoral catheter
Schoonmaker multipurpose catheter
Schultze test
Schumaker aortic clamp
Schwarten balloon dilatation catheter
Schwarten LP guide wire
Schwartz clamp
Sci-Med balloon
Sci-Med SSC "Skinny" catheter
scimitar-shaped flap
scintigram, thallium perfusion
scintigraphy (scintography)
　AMA-Fab (antimyosin monoclonal antibody with Fab fragment)

scintigraphy *(cont.)*
　dipyridamole thallium 201
　dual intracoronary
　exercise thallium
　gated blood pool
　indium-111
　infarct-avid hot-spot
　labeled FFA (free fatty acid)
　microsphere perfusion
　myocardial
　myocardial cold-spot perfusion
　myocardial perfusion
　NEFA (non-esterified fatty acid)
　^{99m}Tc-PYP
　planar thallium
　pulmonary
　pyrophosphate
　thallium-201 myocardial
scintiscan
scissors
　bandage
　Beall circumflex artery
　Church
　coronary artery
　Crafoord thoracic
　curved
　DeBakey endarterectomy
　DeBakey valve
　DeMartel vascular
　Diethrich coronary
　Diethrich valve
　dissecting
　Duffield
　Finochietto thoracic
　Haimovici arteriotomy
　Harrington-Mayo thoracic
　Howell coronary
　iris
　Kantrowitz vascular
　Karmody venous
　Lincoln
　Lincoln-Metzenbaum
　Litwak mitral valve
　Mayo
　Metzenbaum

scissors *(cont.)*
　microvascular
　Mills arteriotomy
　Nelson
　Potts 60° angled
　Potts vascular
　Potts-Smith vascular
　Real coronary artery
　right-angle
　Satinsky
　Smith
　Snowden-Pencer
　Stille-Mayo
　straight
　Strully
　valve
　Willauer thoracic
　Wilmer
SCL (sinus cycle length)
sclerosis, coronary
sclerotic
scope, Jako anterior commissure
score
　Estes EKG
　Gensini coronary artery disease
　mean wall motion
　QRS
　Romhilt-Estes left ventricular
　　hypertrophy
　Selvester QRS
　TAPSE (tricuspid annular plane
　　systolic excursion)
　wall motion
scotoma
scout films
screen, collagen vascular
screw-in lead pacemaker
SCV-CPR (simultaneous compression-ventilation CPR)
SD (standard deviation)
SDPS (protamine solution)
SE (standard error)
sea gull bruit; murmur
seated, valve is
secundum and sinus venosus defects

secundum atrial septal defect
sed (sedimentation) rate
sedentary lifestyle
Seecor pacemaker
seesaw (to-and-fro) murmur
segment
   akinetic
   amplitude and slope of ST
   anterior
   anterobasal
   anterolateral
   apex
   apical
   depressed PR
   depressed ST
   diaphragmatic
   distal
   elevated ST
   hypokinetic
   inferior
   inferoapical
   inferoposterior
   noninfarcted
   posterobasal
   posterolateral
   PR
   proximal
   septal wall
   septum
   ST
   TQ
   upsloping ST
segmental wall motion abnormality
segs (segmented neutrophils)
Seg(s) (segment)(s)
Sehrt clamp
Sehrt compressor
SEI (subendocardial infarction)
Seldinger percutaneous technique
Seldinger technique, modified
selective arteriogram
selective coronary cineangiography
selective visualization
self-retaining retractor
Selman clamp
Selman vessel forceps
Selverstone carotid clamp
Selverstone cardiotomy hook
Selvester QRS score
Semb forceps
Semb lung retractor
Semb rongeur
senescent aortic stenosis
Senn retractor
Senning atrial baffle repair
Senning intra-atrial baffle
Senning procedure for transposition
sensation, pressure-like
sensing
   afterpotential
   pacemaker
   R wave
sensing spike
sensitivity, pacemaker
Sensolog pacemaker
Sensor Kelvin pacemaker
Sensor-Medics metabolic cart
SEP (systolic ejection period)
separation
   aortic cusp
   leaflet
sepsis, catheter-related (CRS)
septal amplitude; thickness
septal arcade
septal collateral
septal defect
septal dip
septal hypoperfusion on thallium
   scan
septal pathway
septal perforator branch
septal separation
septation
septectomy
   atrial
   Blalock-Hanlon atrial
   Blalock-Hanlon partial atrial
septostomy
   balloon atrial
   blade

septostomy *(cont.)*
   blade and balloon atrial
   Mullins transseptal blade and balloon atrial
   Park blade amd balloon atrial
   Rashkind balloon atrial
   Rashkind blade
   Rashkind-Miller atrial
septum
   anteroapical trabecular
   asymmetric hypertrophy of
   atrial
   canal
   dyskinetic
   infundibular
   interatrial (IAS)
   interventricular (IVS)
   membranous
   muscular
   thickened
   ventricular
sequential dilatations
sequential obstruction
sequestered lobe of lung
Sequicor pacemaker
SER (systolic ejection rate)
serial changes
serial EKG tracings
serial electrophysiologic testing (SET)
serial lesions
seriography
seroma, graft
serum electrophoresis
serum iron
serum lipid level
serum lipid profile
serum prothrombin conversion accelerator (SPCA)
sessile plaque
SET (serial electrophysiologic testing)
sewing ring
SF wave of cardiac apex pulse
SFA (superficial femoral artery)

SFHb (stroma-free hemoglobin, pyridoxilated)
SFR (stenotic flow reserve)
SGOT (serum glutamic-oxaloacetic transaminase)
SGPT (serum glutamic-pyruvic transaminase)
shadow
   bat's wing (on x-ray)
   butterfly (on x-ray)
Shapiro sign
sharp waves
shaver catheter
shears
   Bethune rib
   Gluck rib
   Sauerbruch rib
   Shoemaker rib
   Stille-Giertz rib
sheath
   angioplasty
   arterial
   catheter
   check-valve
   Cook transseptal
   Cordis
   femoral artery
   guiding
   introducer
   Mullins
   Mullins transseptal
   peel-away
   tearaway
   transseptal
   USCI angioplasty guiding
   vascular
   venous
sheath and side-arm
sheath with side-arm adapter
sheath-dilator, Mullins transseptal
sheepskin boot
Sheffield exercise test protocol
Sheffield modification of Bruce treadmill protocol
Sheffield treadmill exercise protocol

Sheldon catheter
shell, ejection
shepherd's hook or crook deformity
shift
   ST segment
   superior frontal axis
shift to the left
shift to the right
Shiley guiding catheter
Shiley-Ionescu catheter
Shimazaki area-length method
SHJR4s (side-hole Judkins right, curve 4 French, short) catheter
shock
   cardiogenic
   DC electrical
   diastolic
   hypovolemic
   vasogenic
shock blocks
Shoemaker rib shears
Shone anomaly
short-axis parasternal view
short-axis plane on echocardiography
shortening, mean rate of circumferential
shortness of breath (SOB)
shortwindedness
shoulder of the heart
shudder, carotid
shudder of carotid arterial pulse
shunt
   aorta to pulmonary artery
   aorticopulmonary
   aortopulmonary
   arteriovenous
   ascending aorta to pulmonary artery
   bidirectional
   Blalock
   Blalock-Taussig
   cardiac
   descending thoracic aorta to pulmonary artery

shunt *(cont.)*
   dialysis
   extracardiac
   Glenn
   Gore-Tex
   Gott
   Holter
   intracardiac
   intrapericardial aorticopulmonary
   intrapulmonary
   Javid endarterectomy
   L ► R (left-to-right)
   left-to-right
   modified Blalock-Taussig
   net
   peritoneovenous
   portasystemic vascular
   Potts
   Pruitt-Inahara carotid
   reversed (right-to-left)
   R ► L (right-to-left)
   right-to-left (reversed)
   subclavian artery to pulmonary artery
   systemic-pulmonary artery
   vena cava to pulmonary artery
   Waterston
   Waterston-Cooley
SHU-454 contrast medium
shunted blood
shunting of blood, marked
Shy-Drager syndrome
SI (sinus irregularity; stroke index)
sick sinus syndrome (SSS)
SICOR (computer-assisted cardiac catheter recording system)
side-arm adapter, sheath with
side-arm pressure port
side-biting clamp
side-hole catheter
sidewinder catheter
Siemens electrode
Siemens pacemaker
Siemens-Albis bicycle ergometer
Siemens-Elema pacemaker

Siemens-Elema AB pulse transducer
  probe
Siemens-Pacesetter pacemaker
Siemens PTCA/open heart table
sign
  ace of spades (on angiogram)
  antler (on x-ray)
  Bamberger
  Bouillaud
  Bozzolo
  Branham
  Braunwald
  Broadbent inverted
  Brockenbrough
  Cardarelli
  cardiorespiratory
  Carvallo
  Castellino
  Cegka
  Charcot
  clenched fist
  Corrigan
  cuff
  Delbet
  de Musset
  de Mussy
  Dorendorf
  Drummond
  Duroziez
  E (on x-ray)
  Ebstein
  Ewart
  Federici
  Fischer
  Friedreich
  Glasgow
  gooseneck (on x-ray)
  Grancher
  Greene
  Grocco
  Grossman
  Gunn crossing
  Hall
  Hamman
  Heim-Kreysig

sign *(cont.)*
  Hill
  Homans
  Hope
  Huchard
  Jaccoud
  jugular
  Kussmaul
  Lancisi
  Landolfi
  Levine
  Livierato
  Mahler
  Mannkopf
  McGinn-White
  Meltzer
  Mueller
  Musset
  Osler
  pad
  Perez
  Potain
  Prevel
  Queckenstedt
  Quénu-Muret
  Quincke
  rabbit ear
  reversed-three (on x-ray)
  Rivero-Carvallo
  Robertson
  Rotch
  Sansom
  Shapiro
  Smith
  square root
  Sterles
  trapezius ridge
  Traube
  vein
  wind sock (echocardiogram)
signal-averaged electrocardiogram
  (SAECG)
signif (significant)(ly)
Sigvaris compression stockings
Silastic bead embolization

Silastic catheter
Silastic electrode casing
Silastic H.P. tissue expander
Silastic loop
Silastic tape
Silastic tubing
Silastic vessel loop
silent myocardial infarction; ischemia
silhouette, widened cardiac
Silicore catheter
Silver syndrome
SIMA (single internal mammary artery) reconstruction
Simmons catheter
Simmons-type sidewinder catheter
Simon-Nitlol IVC filter
Simplus catheter
Simplus PE/t dilatation catheter
Simpson atherectomy
Simpson atherectomy device, PET balloon
Simpson peripheral AtheroCath
Simpson rule method for ventricular volume
Simpson Ultra-Low Profile II balloon catheter
Simpson-Robert catheter
Singley forceps
sinoatrial (SA) block; node
sinotubular junction
sinus
   aortic
   aortic valve
   carotid
   coronary (CS)
   distal coronary (DCS)
   left coronary
   middle coronary (MCS)
   noncoronary
   pericardial
   proximal coronary (PCS)
   pulmonary
   transverse
sinus arrest
sinus bradycardia
sinus cycle length (SCL)
sinus exit block
sinus impulse
sinus-initiated QRS complex
sinus irregularity (SI)
sinus mechanism
sinus nodal reentry
sinus node automaticity
sinus node dysfunction
sinus node reentry
sinus of Valsalva
sinus pause
sinus rhythm, normal
sinus segment
sinus slowing
sinus tachycardia
sinus venosus
situs inversus totalis
situs solitus
sizer, prosthetic valve
Sjögren syndrome
skin
   cool and clammy
   diaphoretic
skin wheal
skipping a heartbeat
sl (slight)(ly)
SLE (systemic lupus erythematosus)
sling
   pericardial
   pulmonary artery
SLMD (symptomatic left main disease)
slope
   closing (on echo)
   disappearance
   D to E (of mitral valve)
   E to F (of mitral valve)
   flat diastolic
   flattened E to F
   opening (on echo)
   ST/HR (ST segment/heart rate)
slope of valve opening
sloughing of skin from necrosis

sludging of blood
slush, topical cooling with ice
SMA chemistry panel (SMA-6,
  SMA-12, SMA-17) *may include:*
  albumin
  alkaline phosphatase
  ALT
  AST
  BUN
  calcium
  cholesterol
  creatinine
  glucose
  LDH
  phosphorus
  SGOT
  SGPT
  sodium
  total protein
  triglyceride
  uric acid
Smeloff prosthetic valve
Smeloff-Cutter ball-cage prosthetic
  valve
Smith scissors
smoking, pack-years of cigarette
snap
  mitral opening
  opening (OS)
  valvular
snare, caval
Snowden-Pencer forceps
Snowden-Pencer scissors
snowman appearance of heart
  (on x-ray)
SNRT (sinus node recovery time)
SNRT-CL
snugged down, suture was
SOB (shortness of breath)
sodium content of foods
sodium pertechnetate Tc-99m
SOF-T guide wire
Softip diagnostic catheter
Softouch guiding catheter
Softrac

solution
  albumin
  antibiotic
  cardioplegic
  cold cardioplegic
  cold topical saline
  crystalloid cardioplegic
  dextran, saline, papaverine,
    and heparin
  ECS cardioplegic
  Euro-Collins cooling
  Gey fixative
  hand-agitated
  Hank balanced salt
  heparinized saline
  hyperosmotic
  ice-cold physiologic
  ice slush
  Lugol fixative
  Melrose
  modified Collins
  normal saline (NS)
  papaverine
  Plasmalyte A cardioplegic
  Plegisol cardioplegic
  priming
  saline
  uncrystallized cardioplegic
Sondergaard cleft (interatrial
  groove)
Sones arteriography technique
Sones brachial cutdown technique
Sones Cardio-Marker catheter
Sones catheter
Sones cineangiography technique
Sones guide wire
Sones Hi-Flow catheter
Sones Pistrol catheter
Sones cardiac catheterization
Sones coronary arteriography
Sones coronary cineangiography
Sones selective coronary arteriog-
  raphy
sonicated Renografin-76 contrast
  medium

sonogram, sonography
Sorin pacemaker
Sorin prosthetic valve
SOS guide wire
souffle, mammary (sound on auscultation)
sound, sounds
  A_2 (aortic closure) heart
  adventitious heart
  auscultatory
  bellows
  booming diastolic rumble
  distant heart
  eddy
  ejection
  first heart (S_1)
  fixed splitting of second heart
  flapping
  fourth heart (S_4)
  gallop
  heart
  Korotkoff heart
  M_1 (mitral valve closure) heart
  mammary souffle
  muffled heart
  P_2 (pulmonic closure) heart
  pacemaker heart
  paradoxical splitting of second heart
  paradoxically split S_2 heart
  physiologic heart
  physiologic splitting of second heart
  physiologic third heart
  pericardial friction
  pistol-shot femoral
  prosthetic valve
  pulmonary component of second heart
  reduced
  S_1 (first heart sound)
  S_2 (second heart sound)
  S_3 (third heart sound)
  S_4 (fourth heart sound)
sound *(cont.)*
  sail
  second heart (S_2)
  souffle (heart puffing sound)
  split
  T_1 (tricuspid valve closure) heart
  tambour (drum)
  third heart (S_3)
  tic-tac
  to-and-fro
  tumor plop heart
  weak heart
  widely split second heart
S/P (status post)
space
  antecubital
  echo-free
  epicardial
  fifth intercostal
  His-perivascular
  intercostal
  left fifth intercostal
  left intercostal (LICS)
  pericardial
  perivascular
  pleural
  popliteal
  posterior septal
sparkling appearance of myocardium
spasm
  catheter-induced
  catheter-induced coronary artery
  coronary
  coronary artery (CAS)
  diffuse arteriolar
  postbypass
spatial, two-dimensional
spatula
SPCA (serum prothrombin conversion accelerator)
speckled pattern
SPECT (single photon emission computed tomography)
SPECT thallium scan
SPECT tomography

Spectraflex pacemaker
spectral analysis; pattern
Spectrax programmable Medtronic
  pacemaker
Spectrax SXT pacemaker
Spens syndrome
sphygmography
sphygmomanometer, cuff
spider x-ray view
spike
  atrial
  H and H' (H prime)
  sensing
  wave
spinal needle
spiral dissection
spirometer
  Tissot
  incentive
splinter hemorrhage
splitting of S_1 or S_2
sponge
  4 x 4
  Collostat hemostatic
  laparotomy
  Ray-Tec
  stick
spot
  cold
  hot
  milk
  Roth
spreader
  Bailey rib
  Burford rib
  Burford-Finochietto rib
  Davis rib
  DeBakey rib
  Favalaro-Morse rib
  Finochietto rib
  Haight rib
  Harken rib
  Lemmon sternal
  Lilienthal rib
  Medicon

spreader *(cont.)*
  Miltex rib
  Morse sternal
  Nelson rib
  Rehbein rib
  Reinhoff-Finochietto rib
  Tuffier rib
  Weinberg rib
  Wilson rib
spur, calcific
sputum
  blood-tinged
  frothy
  pink
  rusty
S-QRS interval
squatting to relieve dyspnea
SR (slew rate)
SRT (segmented ring tripolar) lead
SSS (sick sinus syndrome; subclavian steal syndrome)
ST (sinus tachycardia))
ST depression
  downsloping
  horizontal
  reciprocal
ST interval
ST segment
  coved
  depressed
  elevated
  isoelectric
  sagging
  upsloping
ST segment abnormality
ST segment depression, slight
ST segment elevation, marked; slight
ST segment shift
ST segment vector forces
ST vector
ST wave
stab wound, separate
Stack perfusion coronary dilatation catheter

Stage I-VII of Bruce protocol
stain, Gram
stainless steel staples
Stairmaster mobile stairs
standard Bruce protocol
standard deviation (SD)
standard error (SE)
standby pacemaker
standstill
   atrial
   cardiac
   ventricular
Stanford treadmill exercise protocol
Stanicor pacemaker
staphcidal drug
stapler, Auto-Suture surgical
staples, stainless steel
Starling law
Starling mechanism
Starr-Edwards pacemaker
Starr-Edwards aortic valve
   prosthesis
Starr-Edwards ball valve prosthesis
Starr-Edwards disk valve prosthesis
Starr-Edwards mitral prosthesis
Starr-Edwards Silastic valve
stasis, venous
stasis dermatitis
stasis edema
stasis of blood flow
Statham electromagnetic flowmeter
Statham strain-gauge transducer
status, functional
status anginosus
status post (S/P)
steam autoclaved
Steell murmur
steep Trendelenburg position
stellectomy
Stellite ring material of prosthetic
   valve
stenosing ring of left atrium
stenosis
   American Heart Association
     classification of

stenosis *(cont.)*
   aortic (AS)
   aortic valvular
   aortoiliac
   branch pulmonary
   calcific aortic
   calcific bicuspid valvular
   calcific mitral
   calcific senile aortic valvular
   calcific valvular
   carotid artery
   congenital aortic valvular
   congenital mitral
   congenital pulmonary
   congenital tricuspid
   coronary artery
   coronary luminal
   coronary ostial
   critical
   critical coronary
   critical valvular
   discrete subvalvular aortic
     (DSAS)
   dynamic subaortic
   eccentric
   fibromuscular subaortic
   fixed-orifice aortic
   flow limiting
   focal eccentric
   hemodynamically significant
   high-grade
   hypertrophic infundibular sub-
     pulmonic
   idiopathic hypertrophic subaortic
     (IHSS)
   infundibular
   infundibular pulmonic
   innominate artery
   linear
   luminal
   membranous
   mitral (MS)
   mitral valve
   noncalcified
   noncalcified coronary

| stenosis | 153 | stimulation |

stenosis *(cont.)*
  noncritical
  nonrheumatic aortic
  peripheral arterial
  peripheral pulmonary artery (PPAS)
  postangioplasty
  preangioplasty
  pulmonary
  pulmonary artery branch
  pulmonary valve
  pulmonary valvular
  pulmonic (PS)
  renal artery
  rheumatic aortic
  rheumatic aortic valvular
  rheumatic mitral
  rheumatic tricuspid
  segmental
  senescent aortic
  severe
  stenotic
  subaortic
  subpulmonary
  subpulmonic
  subvalvar aortic
  subvalvular aortic
  supra-aortic
  supravalvar aortic
  supravalvular
  supravalvular aortic
  tight
  tricuspid (TS)
  tricuspid valve
  tubular
  unicusp aortic
  valvar aortic
  valvular aortic
  valvular pulmonic
stenosis area
stenosis diameter
stenosis length
stenosis with a spastic component
stenotic coronary artery
stenotic lesion

stent
  activated balloon expandable intravascular
  balloon expandable intravascular
  coil vascular
  Dacron
  endoluminal
  Gianturco
  Medinvent vascular
  Palmaz vascular
  spring-loaded vascular
stepdown unit
stepped-care antihypertensive regimen
stepup, O_2 (or step-up)
Sterles sign
sternal angle of Louis
sternal border, left
sternal splitting
sternal wire
Sternberg myocardial insufficiency
Sternberg pericarditis
sternotomy, median
sternum, burning sensation over
Stertzer brachial guiding catheter
Stertzer-Myler extension wire
stethoscope
  bell of
  diaphragm of
  nuclear
Stewart-Hamilton technique for cardiac output
ST/HR slope (ST segment/heart rate)
STI (systolic time interval)
stick (venipuncture or arterial puncture)
stick tie
stigmata
Still murmur
Stille-Crawford clamp
Stille-Giertz rib shears
Stille-Mayo scissors
stimulation
  atrial single and double extra-

stimulation *(cont.)*
   programmed electrical (PES)
   ventricular single and double extrastimulation threshold of pacemaker
stimuli (pl. of stimulus)
   paired
   premature
stimulator
   Bloom DTU 201 external
   Bloom programmable
stimulus, afterpotential
stippling of lung fields
stitch, anchoring (see *suture*)
St. Jude bi-leaflet prosthetic valve
St. Jude composite valved conduit
St. Jude Medical bi-leaflet valve
St. Jude valve prosthesis
stockings
   antiembolism
   Jobst
   Jobst-Stride support
   Jobst-Stridette support
   Sigvaris compression
   Stride support
   TED (thromboembolic disease)
   Vairox high compression vascular
   VenES II Medical
   Zimmer antiembolism support
Stokes-Adams attack; disease
Stokes-Adams syndrome
stoma, coronary artery
stone heart
Storz needle cannula
straight AP pelvic injection
straight flush percutaneous catheter
strain
   left ventricular (LV)
   right ventricular (RV)
strain-gauge, mercury-in-Silastic
strain pattern on EKG
strep throat
streptococcal sore throat
streptococcus, group A
Streptococcus pyogenes

stress-induced
stress management
stress thallium scan
stress thallium-201 myocardial imaging
Stride support stockings
strip
   cardiac monitor
   EKG monitor
   felt
   rhythm
   transtelephonic rhythm
stripper
   Alexander rib
   Babcock vein
   Dunlop thrombus
   Emerson vein
   endarterectomy
   external vein
   internal vein
   Matson rib
   Mayo vein
   Meyer vein
   Nabatoff vein
   olive-tipped
   Trace vein
   vein
   Webb vein
stripper with bullet end
stripping, varicose vein
stripping of multiple communicators
stripping of perforators and communicators
stroke, thromboembolic (TE)
stroke ejection rate
stroke index (SI)
stroke power
stroke volume (SV)
stroke work
Strully scissors
strut
   tricuspid valve
   valve outflow
Stryker saw
Stuart blood coagulation factor

Stuart-Prower blood coagulation
    factor
study
    cardiac wall motion
    Doppler flow
    electrophysiologic (EP)
    enzyme
    first-pass
    Framingham
    gated blood pool
    periorbital Doppler
    wall motion
stump pressure
stylet
    straight
    transseptal
ST segment depression
    downsloping
    exercise-induced
    horizontal
    reciprocal
    upsloping
ST segment displacement
ST segment elevation
ST segment shift
ST and T wave changes
sub (subendocardial)
subannular region
subclavian approach for cardiac
    catheterization
subclavian peel-away sheath
subclavian steal syndrome (SSS)
subcostal
subcostal approach
subcutaneous pocket
subcutaneous tunnel
subendocardial infarction (SEI)
subendocardial myocardial infarction
subendocardial resection
subfascially
sublingual nitroglycerin
suboptimal visualization
suboptimally visualized
subpectoral implantation of pulse
    generator

Subramanian clamp
substernal
subvalvular
subxiphoid approach
subxiphoid echocardiography view
Sucquet-Hoyer anastomosis
sudden cardiac death
suffocating chest pain
Sugiura vascular surgery procedure
    for esophageal varices
sulcus
    atrioventricular
    pulmonary
sulcus terminalis
sulfur colloid, technetium bound to
SULP II catheter
Sumida cardioangioscope
summation gallop (S_3 and S_4)
summit, ventricular septal
sump
sump pump
Sundt-Kees clip for aneurysms
superficial femoral artery occlusion
superior vena cava syndrome
SuperStat hemostatic agent
supersystemic pulmonary artery
    pressure
suppression of arrhythmia
supra-annular constriction
supra-annular suture ring
supra-aortic ridge
supraceliac aorta
supracristal ventricular septal defect
supra-Hisian block
suprasternal notch view on echo-
    cardiogram
supravalvar aortic stenosis
    syndrome
supravalvular aortic stenosis
supravalvular aortogram
supraventricular crest
supraventricular ectopic levels
supraventricular tachycardia (SVT),
    inducible sustained orthodromic
surgery (see *operation)*

surgical field
surgical intervention
Surgical Nu-Knit
surgical revascularization
Surgicel gauze
Surgilene suture
Surgitool 200 prosthetic valve
sustained or nonsustained reciprocating tachycardia
Sutter-Smeloff heart valve prosthesis
suture
  absorbable
  anchoring
  angle
  atraumatic
  black
  braided silk
  bridle
  buried
  catgut
  chromic
  chromic catgut
  circular
  coated
  collagen
  continuous
  cotton
  Dacron
  Dacron-bolstered
  deep
  Deklene
  Dermalene
  Dermalon
  Dexon
  Dexon Plus
  double-armed
  doubly ligated
  dural tenting
  EPTFE (expanded polytetrafluoroethylene) vascular
  Ethibond
  Ethicon
  Ethiflex
  Ethilon

suture *(cont.)*
  figure-of-8
  Flexon steel
  Gregory stay
  gut
  heavy silk
  heavy wire
  horizontal
  horizontal mattress
  imbricating
  intermittent
  interrupted
  intracuticular
  inverted
  inverting
  Lembert
  ligature
  locked
  locking
  loop
  mattress
  Maxon
  Mersilene
  monofilament absorbable
  monofilament nylon
  nonabsorbable
  noneverting
  Novofil
  Nurolon
  nylon
  over-and-over whip
  patch-reinforced mattress
  pericostal
  Perma-Hand
  plain
  plastic
  pledgeted
  pledgeted Ethibond
  Polydek
  polypropylene
  pop-off
  Potts tie
  preplaced
  Prolene
  pursestring or purse-string

suture *(cont.)*
  reabsorbable
  retention
  running
  seromuscular-to-edge
  silk
  simple
  single-armed
  skin staples
  stainless steel wire
  staples
  Steri-Strips
  stitch
  subcutaneous
  subcuticular
  Surgilene
  synthetic
  Teflon
  Teflon-pledgeted
  tenting
  Tevdek pledgeted
  through-and-through continuous
  Ti-Cron
  traction
  transfixion
  Trumbull
  Tycron
  U double-barrel
  umbilical tape
  undyed
  vertical
  Vicryl
  whipstitch
  white
  wire
suture ligature
SV (stroke volume)
SVC (superior vena cava)
SVG (saphenous vein graft)
SVI (stroke volume index)
SVPC (supraventricular premature contraction)
SVR (systemic vascular resistance)
SVT (supraventricular tachycardia)
Swan aortic clamp

Swan-Ganz balloon-flotation catheter
Swan-Ganz catheter
Swan-Ganz Guidewire TD catheter
Swan-Ganz pulmonary artery catheter
Swan-Ganz technique for cardiac catheterization
Swan-Ganz thermodilution catheter
Sweet sternal punch
swelling, ankle
SWI (stroke work index)
Sydenham chorea
Symbion pneumatic assist device
Symbios pacemaker
sympathectomy
  high thoracic left
  lumbar
  regional cardiac
symphysis pubis
symptom-limited exercise test
symptom reproduced with exertion
symptomatic digitalis-induced bradyarrhythmia
synchronized DC cardioversion
synchronous mode of pacemaker
synchrony, atrioventricular
syncopal attack
syncope
  Adams-Stokes
  cardiac
  cardiogenic
  carotid sinus
  cerebrovascular
  cough
  exertional
  glossopharyngeal-vagal
  micturition
  near
  orthostatic
  positional
  pressor-postpressor
  tussive
  vasovagal
  X

syndrome
  Adams-Stokes
  angina with normal coronaries
  anomalous first thoracic rib
  aortic arch
  apical systolic click-murmur
  atypical chest pain
  Ayerza
  Barlow
  Bernheim
  Blackfan-Diamond
  blue finger
  blue toe ("trash foot")
  Bouillaud
  Bradbury-Eggleston
  bradycardia-tachycardia
  bradytachycardia
  bradytachydysrhythmia
  carotid sinus (CSS)
  Charcot-Weiss-Baker
  CHARGE
  Chiari-Budd
  chronic hyperventilation
  click
  click-murmur
  compartment
  concealed Wolff-Parkinson-White
  coronary steal
  costoclavicular
  CREST
  DaCosta
  declamping shock
  de Lange
  DiGeorge
  Down
  Dressler
  Dysshwannian
  effort
  Ehlers-Danlos
  Eisenmenger
  elfin facies
  Ellis-van Creveld
  external carotid steal
  fibrinogen-fibrin conversion
  flapping valve

syndrome *(cont.)*
  floppy valve
  Forrester
  gastrocardiac
  Goldenhar
  Hamman-Rich
  Hegglin
  hemañgioma-thrombocytopenia
  hemopleuropneumonia
  holiday heart
  Holt-Oram
  hyperkinetic heart
  hypersensitive carotid sinus
  hyperviscosity
  hypoplastic left-heart (HLHS)
  hypoplastic right-heart
  idiopathic long QT interval
  intermediate coronary
  ischemic heart disease
  Ivemark
  Jervell and Lange-Nielsen
  Kartagener
  Kasabach-Merritt
  Kawasaki
  Klein-Waardenburg
  Klippel-Feil
  Kussmaul
  Laurence-Moon-Biedl
  Leriche
  Lev
  LGL (Lown-Ganong-Levine)
    variant
  Libman-Sacks
  long QT (LQTS)
  long QT$_c$ interval
  Lown-Ganong-Levine (LGL)
  Lutembacher
  Marfan
  Martorell
  Ménière
  mitral valve prolapse
  Moynahan
  Noonan
  P mitrale
  P pulmonale

syndrome *(cont.)*
  pacemaker
  paraneoplastic
  pericardiotomy
  Pick
  Polhemus-Schafer-Ivemark
  postcardiotomy psychosis
  postcommissurotomy
  postmyocardial infarction
  postpericardiotomy
  postphlebitic
  post-thrombotic
  preexcitation
  preinfarction
  primary mitral valve prolapse
  prolonged QT interval
  pseudoclaudication
  QT
  Raynaud
  Romano-Ward
  Rosenbach
  Rubenstein-Taybi
  Sanchez-Cascos cardioauditory
  scalenus anticus
  Scheie
  scimitar
  shoulder-hand
  Shy-Drager
  sick sinus (SSS)
  Silver
  Sjögren
  Spens
  splenic flexure
  stiff heart
  Stokes-Adams
  subclavian steal (SSS)
  superficial vena cava
  superior vena cava
  supravalvar aortic stenosis
  supravalvular aortic stenosis
  surdocardiac
  Swan-Ganz
  systolic click-late systolic
      murmur
  tachycardia-bradycardia

syndrome *(cont.)*
  Takayasu
  Taussig-Bing
  thoracic outlet
  thoracic outlet compression
  thrombocytopenia-absent radius
      (TAR)
  thromboembolic
  trash foot
  trisomy 13; 21
  Trousseau
  twiddler's
  vascular
  vena cava
  von Willebrand
  Waardenburg
  Ward-Romano
  Williams
  Wolff-Parkinson-White (WPW)
syndrome X
Synergyst DDD pacemaker
Synthaderm dressing
system
  CASE computerized exercise EKG
  Cenflex central monitoring
  conduction
  COROSKOP C cardiac imaging
  CGR biplane angiographic
  Desilets introducer
  dominant left coronary artery
  Echovar Doppler
  Frank XYZ orthogonal lead
  Haemonetics Cell-Saver
  His-Purkinje (HPS)
  Hombach lead placement
  Innovator Holter
  kallikrein-kinin
  Mason-Likar 12-lead ECG
  MEDDARS cardiac catheteriza-
      tion analysis
  Novacore left ventricular assist
      (LVAS)
  pacemaker tester
  Probe balloon-on-a-wire dilata-
      tion

system *(cont.)*
    Q-cath catheterization recording
    Quinton computerized exercise EKG
    Rozanski lead placement
    SICOR (computer-assisted cardiac catheter recording)
    single-chamber cardiac pacing (PASYS)
    Thora-Klex chest drainage
    TRON 3 VACI cardiac imaging
    USCI Probe balloon-on-a-wire dilatation
    V_1-like ambulatory lead
    V_5-like ambulatory lead
    Viagraph computerized exercise EKG
    water-seal drainage
System, Haemonetics Cell Saver
System, Medtronic Interactive Tachycardia Terminating
systemic AV O_2 difference
systemic pressure
systemic resistance
systemic and topical hypothermia
systemic vascular resistance (SVR)
systole
    aborted
    atrial
    cardiac
    coupled premature
    extra
    frustrate
    premature atrial
    premature junctional
    premature ventricular
    total
    ventricular
    ventricular ectopic
systolic anterior motion (SAM) of mitral valve
systolic click
systolic/diastolic blood pressure
systolic ejection murmur
systolic ejection period (SEP)
systolic fractional shortening
systolic pressure
systolic trough
systolic upstroke time

T

T artifact
T/D ratio (thickness to diameter of ventricle)
T loop
T-Span tissue expander
T vector
T wave
    biphasic
    depressed
    diphasic
    enlarged
    flattened
    flipped
    hyperacute

T wave *(cont.)*
    inverted
    ischemic
    pseudonormalization of inverted
    tall
    upright
T wave amplitude, increased
T wave changes
T wave flattening
T wave inversion, terminal
T_1 heart sound (tricuspid valve closure)
Tc myocardial imaging
Ta wave

TA-55 stapling device
table
  anterior
  posterior
  Siemens PTCA/open heart
table of the sternum
TAC atherectomy catheter
tachyarrhythmia
  atrial
  digitalis-induced
  drug-resistant
  ectopic
  paroxysmal
  paroxysmal ventricular
  sustained ventricular
  ventricular
tachycardia
  accelerated idioventricular
  antidromic
  antidromic AV reentrant
  antidromic circus-movement
  antidromic reciprocating
  atrial
  atrial automatic
  atrial paroxysmal (APT)
  atrial reentrant
  atrial reentry
  atrioventricular nodal (AVNT)
  atrioventricular nodal reentrant (AVNRT)
  atrioventricular reciprocating (AVRT)
  atypical AV nodal reentry
  automatic atrial
  automatic ectopic (AET)
  AV nodal reentry
  AV reciprocating
  benign ventricular
  bidirectional ventricular
  bundle branch block (BBB)
  chaotic atrial
  circus-movement (CMT)
  concealed accessory pathway (AP)
  concealed bypass-type

tachycardia *cont.)*
  double
  drug-refractory
  ectopic atrial
  ectopic supraventricular
  endless-loop
  exercise-aggravated ventricular
  exercise-induced ventricular
  fast-slow AV nodal reentrant
  focal ventricular
  hypokalemia-induced ventricular
  idioventricular
  incessant ectopic atrial
  incessant focal atrial
  inducible
  intra-atrial reentrant
  intractable ventricular
  junctional
  malignant ventricular
  monomorphic
  monomorphic ventricular
  multifocal atrial (MAT or MFAT)
  multiform
  narrow-complex
  nodal reentrant
  nodoventricular
  nonparoxysmal AV junctional
  nonparoxysmal junctional
  nonparoxysmal reciprocating junctional (NPRJT)
  nonsustained ventricular
  NPJT (nonparoxysmal AV junctional)
  orthodromic AV reentrant
  orthodromic reciprocating (ORT)
  orthodromic supraventricular
  orthostatic
  pacemaker-mediated
  parasystolic ventricular
  paroxysmal atrial (PAT)
  paroxysmal junctional (PJT)
  paroxysmal sinus
  paroxysmal supraventricular (PSVT)

tachycardia *(cont.)*
  pleomorphic
  polymorphic ventricular
  rapid nonsustained ventricular
  reciprocating
  reentrant
  reflex
  refractory
  repetitive monomorphic ventricular (RMVT)
  repetitive paroxysmal ventricular
  resting
  runs of
  SA nodal reentry
  self-terminating
  sinoatrial (SA) reentrant
  sinus
  sinus reentrant
  slow retrograde
  slow-fast
  slow-fast AV nodal reentrant
  supraventricular (SVT)
  sustained ventricular
  ventricular (VT)
  wide QRS
  wide-complex
  Wolff-Parkinson-White reentrant
  WPW (Wolff-Parkinson-White)
tachydysrhythmia
Tachylog pacemaker
tachypnea
TAD guide wire
tag, epicardial fat
TAH (total artificial heart)
Takayasu aortitis
Takayasu arteritis
Takayasu disease; syndrome
takeoff of vessel
taking down of adhesions
tambour sound
tamponade
  cardiac
  chronic
  pericardial

tape
  compression
  Dacron
  Silastic
  umbilical
  vascular
TAPSE (tricuspid annular plane systolic excursion) score
TAPVC (total anomalous pulmonary venous connection)
TAPVR (total anomalous pulmonary venous return)
TAR (thrombocytopenia-absent radius) syndrome
tardus et parvus, pulsus
target heart rate
Tascon prosthetic valve
Taussig-Bing congenital anomaly of heart
Taussig-Bing syndrome
TAV (transcutaneous aorto-velography)
Tawara, node of
Tc-99m pyrophosphate
TCBF (total cerebral blood flow)
TE (thromboembolic) stroke
tearaway sheath
teased off
TEB (thoracic electrical bio-impedance)
TEC (transluminal extraction catheter)
technetium bound to DTPA
technetium bound to serum albumin
technetium bound to sulfur colloid
technetium-99m labeled fibrinogen
technetium-99m labeled red blood cells (RBC)
technetium-99m pyrophosphate myocardial imaging; scan
technetium-99m radioisotope
technetium-99m sodium pertechnetate

technician, pump
technique (see also *operation*)
   anterior sandwich patch closure
   Bentall inclusion
   button
   Dotter-Judkins
   dye dilution
   ECG signal-averaging
   extrastimulus
   first-pass
   flow mapping
   gated
   Gruentzig PTCA
   indicator-dilution
   Judkins cardiac catheterization
   Judkins femoral catheterization
   J loop (on catheterization)
   kissing balloon
   Lown
   modified Seldinger
   Mullins blade
   multiple chord, center line echocardiogram
   noninvasive
   percutaneous Judkins
   percutaneous puncture
   percutaneous transfemoral
   PICSO (pressure-controlled intermittent coronary occlusion)
   pressure half-time
   Schonander
   Seldinger percutaneous
   Sones arteriography
   Sones brachial cutdown
   Sones cardiac catheterization
   Sones cineangiography
   Sones coronary arteriography
   Stewart-Hamilton cardiac output
   thermal dilution
   Trusler aortic valve
   upgated
   TED (thromboembolic disease) antiembolism stockings
   TEE (transesophageal echocardiography)

Teflon Bardic plug
Teflon catheter
Teflon felt bolster
Teflon felt pledget
Teflon graft
Teflon intracardiac patch
Teflon patch
Teflon pledget
Teflon-pledgeted suture
Teflon suture
Teichholz equation for left ventricular volume
Tektronix oscilloscope
Telectronics pacing lead
Telectronics pacemaker electrode
Telectronics PASAR antitachycardia pulse generator
telemetry
telephone monitoring of EKG
telephone transmission of EKG
temperature
   core
   esophageal
temporary atrial pacing wire
temporary pacing catheter
tenderness, chest wall
tendon, left ventricular false
tendon of Krehl
tendon of Todaro
Tennis Racquet angiography catheter
tension-time index (TTI)
tensionless anastomosis
tented up
teratogenicity
terminal inversion
terminal negativity of P wave
test
   ^{11}C-palmitate uptake
   ^{11}C-propranolol uptake
   ^{123}I-heptadecanoic acid uptake
   Adson
   Allen
   ANA (antinuclear antibody)
   Anderson-Keys total serum cholesterol

test *(cont.)*
 antihyaluronidase
 antistreptolysin-O titer
 antistreptozyme (ASTZ)
 Apt
 APTT clotting
 ASO titer
 ASTZ (antistreptozyme)
 atrial pacing
 bicycle ergometer
 bicycle exercise
 blood culture
 cardiokymographic (CKG)
 carotid sinus
 cold pressor (Hines and Brown)
 cold pressor exercise
 collagen vascular screen
 collateral circulation
 Coombs
 costoclavicular
 Crampton
 cuff
 Dehio
 dehydrocholate
 diaphragmatic stimulation
 dipyridamole echocardiography
 dipyridamole handgrip
 dipyridamole infusion
 direct Coombs
 Duke
 dynamic exercise
 electrophysiologic
 equivocal exercise
 ergonovine provocative
 erythrocyte sedimentation rate (ESR)
 euglobulin lysis
 exercise
 exercise stress
 exercise thallium-201 stress
 exercise tolerance (ETT)
 flat-hand
 Gibbon and Landis
 Goethlin
 graded exercise tolerance

test *(cont.)*
 graded treadmill
 handgrip exercise
 handgrip stress
 Henle-Coenen
 Hess capillary
 Hines and Brown
 Howell
 hydrogen
 hyperabduction
 hyperemia
 hyperventilation
 indirect Coombs
 isometric exercise
 isometric stress
 Korotkoff
 Lewis and Pickering
 Liebermann-Burchard
 Master two-step (2-step) exercise
 Matas
 Moschcowitz
 Newman-Keuls
 noninvasive
 pacemaker threshold
 Pachon
 passive tilt
 Perthes
 Phalen stress
 plantar ischemic
 plasma renin activity (PRA)
 Plesch
 postmyocardial infarction exercise
 primed lymphocyte (PLT)
 prothrombin-proconvertin
 provocative
 PT/PTT
 Quick
 R-lactate enzymatic monotest
 Salkowski
 scalene
 Schiff
 Schultze
 sickle cell
 stress

test *(cont.)*
  submaximal treadmill exercise
  symptom-limited maximal exercise
  teichoic acid antibody
  thallium stress
  thallium-201 exercise
  tilt
  tourniquet
  treadmill exercise (TET)
  treadmill stress (TMST)
  treadmill (TMT)
  Tris-buffer infusion
  Tuffier
  von Recklinghausen
  Zwenger
testing
  extrastimulus (EST)
  serial electrophysiologic (SET)
TET (treadmill exercise test)
tet (tetralogy of Fallot) spells
tetralogy of Fallot (TOF)
  atypical
  pink
tetralogy of Fallot plus atrial septal defect
Tevdek suture
TGA (transposition of great arteries)
thallium, regional myocardial uptake of
thallium clearance
thallium imaging
thallium injection
thallium-201 myocardial imaging
thallium-201 myocardial scintigraphy
thallium myocardial perfusion imaging
thallium perfusion study
thallium stress test
thallium treadmill
thallium uptake
thallium washout
thallous chloride
thebesian foramen

thebesian valve
thebesian vein
Theden method
theorem
  Bayes
  Bernoulli
therapeutic blood level of drug
therapy
  antianginal
  antihypertensive
  diuretic
  quinidine
  step-care hypertensive
  thrombolytic
  transfusion
thermal dilution technique
thermistor catheter
thermistor electrode
thermistor plethysmography
thermodilution balloon catheter
thermodilution cardiac output
thermodilution catheter
thermodilution ejection fraction
thermodilution method for measuring cardiac output
thermodilution Swan-Ganz catheter
thermodilution technique
Thermos pacemaker
THI needle
thickened mitral valve
thickened valvular leaflets
thickening of valve
thickening of valve leaflets
thickening of ventricular wall
thickness
  interventricular septal (IVST)
  IVS wall
  posterior LV wall
  posterior wall (PWT)
  septal
Thomas Allis forceps
Thompson carotid artery clamp
thoracic inlet
thoracic outlet compression syndrome

thoracicoabdominal incision
thoracoplasty, Schede
thoracotomy
  anterolateral
  left lateral
  posterolateral
Thora-Klex chest drainage system
Thoratec BVAD (biventricular assist device)
Thoratec RVAD (right ventricular assist device)
Thoratec VAD (ventricular assist device)
Thorel pathway
Thorotrast contrast medium
three-block claudication
three-vessel coronary disease
threshold
  defibrillation (DFT)
  lead
  myocardial
  pacemaker stimulation
  pacing
  stimulation
threshold current
threshold for arrhythmia
threshold of activation
thrill
  aneurysmal
  aortic
  apical
  basal precordial
  dense
  diastolic
  diastolic apical
  faint
  parasternal systolic
  precordial
  presystolic
  purring
  supramanubrium systolic
  systolic
  vibratory
thrombin, topical
Thrombinar

thromboangiitis obliterans
thromboatherosclerotic process
thrombocytopenia-absent radius syndrome (TAR)
thromboembolectomy
thromboembolism
  aortic
  catheter-induced
  pulmonary
  venous
thromboendarterectomy
  aortoiliofemoral
  carotid
  femoral
thrombolysis, intracoronary
thrombolytic agent; drug; therapy
thrombo-obliterative process
thrombophlebitis, migratory
thrombosis
  agonal
  arterial
  cavernous sinus
  coronary
  coronary artery
  creeping
  deep venous (DVT)
  dilatation
  marasmic
  mesenteric
  postoperative
  propagating
  puerperal
  pulmonary artery
  Ribberts
  superficial venous
  traumatic
  venous
Thrombostat
thrombotic thrombocytopenic purpura
thromboxane A_2
thrombus
  agonal
  annular
  antemortem

thrombus *(cont.)*
  apical
  ball
  blood platelet
  coral
  currant jelly
  hyaline
  intracardiac
  intravascular
  laminated
  luminal
  marasmic
  migratory
  mixed
  mural
  nonocclusive luminal
  obstructive
  occlusive
  organized
  parietal
  pedunculated
  propagating
  red
  saddle
  stratified
  white
thrombus stripper, Dunlop
Thruflex balloon catheter
Thruflex PTCA balloon catheter
thrust
  cardiac
  double systolic outward
  presystolic outward
thump, precordial
thumping of heart in chest
thumpversion (striking patient's chest)
thyroid studies
TI (tricuspid insufficiency) myocardial imaging
TIA (transient ischemic attack)
tibial-peroneal trunk
Ti-Cron suture (also Tycron)
tidal wave of carotid arterial pulse
tie, plastic
tie gun
tightener, wire
time
  acceleration
  activated partial thromboplastin (APTT)
  aortic ischemic
  atrial activation
  atrioventricular
  carotid ejection
  conduction
  corrected sinus node recovery (CSNRT)
  cross-clamp
  deceleration
  donor heart-lung
  donor organ ischemic
  Duke bleeding
  ejection (ET)
  isovolumic contraction
  isovolumic relaxation (IVRT)
  Ivy bleeding
  left ventricular ejection (LVET)
  maximum inflation
  maximum walking (MWT)
  mean pulmonary transit (MTT)
  myocardial contrast appearance (MCAT)
  pain-free walking (PFWT) (on treadmill)
  partial thromboplastin (PTT)
  prothrombin (PT)
  pulmonary transit (PTT)
  pump
  reaction recovery
  sinoatrial conduction (SACT)
  sinus node recovery (SNRT)
  systolic upstroke
  total cross-clamp
  total ischemic
  venous filling (VFT)
  venous return (VRT)
  ventricular activation (VAT)
  ventricular isovolumic relaxation
time activity curve of contrast agent

time-out, ventriculoatrial
time-to-peak contrast (TPC)
time-to-peak filling rate (TPFR)
TIMI (thrombolysis in myocardial
   infarction) classification
TIMI II protocol
TIMI grading system for patency
tin pyrophosphate
tined lead pacemaker
tip
   Andrews suction
   catheter
   Frazier suction
   leaflet
   mitral valve leaflet
   tonsil suction
   valve
   Yankauer suction
Tissot spirometer
tissue
   cryopreserved homograft
   devitalized
tissue expander
   PMT AccuSpan
   Silastic H.P.
   T-Span
tissue perfusion
tissue plasminogen activator (t-PA)
tissue viability
titer, antistreptolysin-O (ASO)
titration of dosage
Titrator
TKO (to keep open), intravenous
Tl (thallium)
TMST (treadmill stress test)
TMT (treadmill test)
to-and-fro murmur
Todaro
   tendon of
   triangle of
Todd units for ASO titer
toenails, thickened
TOF (tetralogy of Fallot)
toilet, pulmonary

tomography
   biplanar cardiac blood pool
   computerized axial (CAT)
   positron emission (PET)
   rapid acquisition computed axial
      (RACAT)
   seven-pinhole
   single photon emission computed
      (SPECT)
   slant-hole
   SPECT (single photon emission
      computed)
tongue
   chicken heart
   geographic
tongue of vein material
top normal limits in size
topical cold saline
topical cooling of heart with saline
topical cooling with ice slush
topical ice
topical lavage
topical myocardial hypothermia
topically cooled
Torcon NB selective angiographic
   catheter
torr
torr pressure
torsade de pointes
tortuosity of blood vessel
tortuosity of superficial veins
tortuous aorta
tortuous vessel
torus aorticus
Toshiba echocardiograph machine
total anomalous pulmonary venous
   drainage; return
total peripheral resistance (TPR)
tour de force
tourniquet
   Medi-Quet surgical
   rotating
   Rumel
   Rumel myocardial

toxicity, digitalis
TP segment on EKG
TPA (thrombotic pulmonary arteriopathy)
t-PA (tissue plasminogen activator)
TPC (time-to-peak contrast) (myocardial)
TPFR (time to peak filling rate)
TPR (temperature, pulse, and respiration; total peripheral resistance; total pulmonary resistance
TQ segment
TR (tricuspid regurgitation)
trabeculae carneae
trabeculation
trace edema
Trace vein stripper
tracer (see *radioisotope)*
tracer activity
tracer dose
tracheal bronchial lavage
tracing
   monitor lead
   postexercise
track valve
tract
   aberrant AV bypass
   atriofascicular
   atriofascicular bypass
   atrio-His
   atrio-Hisian bypass
   atrionodal bypass
   Breckenmacher
   bypass
   fasciculoventricular bypass
   inflow
   internodal
   James atrionodal bypass
   James intranodal
   left ventricular outflow (LVOT)
   left ventricular inflow
   nodoventricular bypass
   outflow
   pulmonary conduit outflow

tract *(cont.)*
   pulmonary outflow
   right ventricular inflow
   right ventricular outflow (RVOT)
   ventricular flow
   ventricular outflow
transaortic gradient
transatrial surgical approach
transcatheter His bundle ablation
transcutaneous femoral artery puncture
transdermal nitroglycerin
transdiaphragmatic approach
transducer
   arterial line
   Bentley
   Diasonics
   epicardial Doppler flow
   Gould Statham pressure
   Hewlett-Packard
   Millar catheter-tip
   M-mode
   pressure
   Statham
   Statham strain-gauge
   strain-gauge
   Ultramark 8
transect, transected, transection
transection of aorta
transesophageal Doppler color flow imaging
transesophageal echocardiography (TEE)
transesophageal pacing
transfixion suture
transfusion, autologous
transfusion therapy
transient ischemic attack (TIA)
transient perfusion defect
transition zone
translingual nitroglycerin
translocation of coronary arteries
transluminal
   transluminal coronary artery angioplasty complex

transluminal extraction catheter (TEC)
transmediastinal pacemaker electrode insertion
transmitral flow
transmucosal nitroglycerin
transmural myocardial infarction
transplant, transplantation
  cardiac
  heart
  heart-lung
  heterotopic
  Lower-Shumway cardiac
  orthotopic cardiac
  syngenesioplastic
transposition
  carotid-subclavian
  Mustard procedure for
  Senning procedure for
transposition of great arteries (TGA)
  complete
  corrected (CTGA)
transposition of great vessels
transposition of pulmonary veins
transpulmonic gradient
Trans-Scan
transseptal approach
transseptal left heart catheterization
transstenotic pressure gradient
transthoracic pacemaker electrode insertion
transvenous ventricular demand pacemaker
transxiphoid approach for pacemaker lead
"trash foot" (blue toe syndrome)
Traube murmur; sign
treadmill
  Astrand
  Borg exertion scale on
  Ellestad
  exercise
  motorized
  Q-Stress

treadmill exercise stress test
treadmill exercise test (TET)
treadmill inclination, incremental increases in
treadmill slope
treadmill speed, incremental increases in
treadmill stress test (TMST)
Tredex powered bicycle
tree-in-winter appearance (on x-ray)
trendscriber
triangle
  Burger scalene
  cardiohepatic
  carotid
  Einthoven
  femoral
  Gerhardt
  Koch
  Todaro
tributary, tributaries
Trichinella myocarditis
tricuspid aortic valve
tricuspid valve (TV)
tricuspid valve annuloplasty
trifascicular block
trifurcation
trigeminal pattern
trigeminy
triglyceride, serum
trigone, fibrous
trigonum caroticum
trileaflet
trimmed on the bias
Trios M pacemaker
triphasic contour of QRS complex
triple-lumen line
triplet
trivial mitral regurgitation
trocar
  Davidson thoracic
  Hurwitz thoracic
  Nelson thoracic
TRON 3 VACI cardiac imaging system

trough, systolic
trough level of drug
Trousseau syndrome
Trousers, Medical Anti-Shock (MAST)
truncated atrial appendage
truncus arteriosus
  common
  persistent
trunk
  brachiocephalic
  common
  peroneal-tibial
  pulmonary
  saphenous
  single arterial
  tibial-peroneal
  twin
trunk of atrioventricular bundle
Trusler technique to reconstruct aortic valve
TS (tricuspid stenosis)
TSV (total stroke volume)
TTI (tension-time index)
TTM (transtelephonic electrocardiogram monitoring)
TU wave
Tubbs mitral valve dilator
tube
  Andrews Pynchon suction
  angled 24F pleural
  Argyle Sentinel Seal chest
  bilateral pleural
  Bivona tracheostomy
  Broncho-Cath endotracheal
  chest
  cuffed endotracheal
  double-lumen endobronchial
  endotracheal
  Endotrol tracheal

tube *(cont.)*
  fenestrated
  Frazier suction
  Hi-Lo Jet tracheal
  Holter
  Lindholm tracheal
  Lo-Pro tracheal
  pleural
  Pleur-evac suction
  polyethylene
  Rehfuss
  right-angle chest
  rubber
  Sarns intracardiac suction
  Silastic
  straight chest
  suction
  Thora-Klex chest
  water-seal chest
  Yankauer suction
tube graft (see *graft)*
tubing (see *tube)*
tubular segment
Tuffier rib spreader
Tuffier test
tumor plop sound
tunnel (verb)
tunnel
  aortico-left ventricular
  aortopulmonary
Tuohy-Bost introducer
turbulence, turbulent
Tuttle thoracic forceps
TV (tricuspid valve)
twin trunk
Tycron suture (also Ti-Cron)
Tygon catheter
type A behavior; personality
type B personality

U

U loop
U wave
U wave inversion
UCG (ultrasonic cardiography)
Uhl anomaly
ulcer
   atheromatous
   heel
   hypertensive ischemic
   ischemic skin
   stasis
   toe
   varicose
   venous
   venous stasis
ulceration
   arteriolar ischemic
   ischemic
ULP (ultra low profile) catheter
Ultracor prosthetic valve
Ultramark 8 transducer
ultrasonic cardiogram (UCG)
ultrasonography, duplex B-mode
ultrasound
   B-mode
   Doppler
   gray-scale
   Hewlett-Packard
   Irex Exemplar
   real-time
   transthoracic
   VingMed
Ultravist contrast medium
umbilical artery
umbilical tape
umbilical vein graft, modified
   human
umbrella, Mobin-Uddin
umbrella filter
underdrive termination
underloading, ventricular
undersensing of pacemaker

unicommissural aortic valve
unifocal
unilateral aortofemoral graft
Unilith pacemaker
unipolar limb lead
unipolar pacemaker
unit
   acute coronary care
   BICAP
   coronary care (CCU)
   critical care (CCU)
   stepdown
   Wood
univentricular heart
Unna boot
unoxygenated blood
unroof, unroofed
upper lobe vein prominence on
   chest x-ray
upright T wave
upright U wave
upsloping ST segment depression
unstable angina
upstream sampling method
upstroke, brisk carotid
uptake (see also *radioisotope*)
   C-11 palmitate
   diffuse myocardial
   increased lung
   increased RV
   localized myocardial
   observed maximal oxygen
   predicted maximal oxygen
Urografin-76 contrast medium
USAFSAM treadmill exercise
   protocol
USCI angioplasty guiding sheath
USCI angioplasty Y connector
USCI arterial sheath
USCI Bard catheter
USCI catheter
USCI guide wire

| USCI | 173 | valve |

USCI guiding catheter
USCI Mini-Profile balloon dilatation catheter
USCI Probe balloon-on-a-wire dilatation system
USCI Sauvage EXS side-limb prosthesis
USCI sheath
Utah TAH (total artificial heart)

V

V (ventricular)
V_1 - V_6 (precordial EKG leads)
V_2A_2 curve
V_1V_2 curve
V_1-like ambulatory lead system
V_5-like ambulatory lead system
V fib (ventricular fibrillation)
V peak of jugular venous pulse
V tach (ventricular tachycardia)
V wave of jugular venous pulse
V wave of right atrial pressure
V wave pressure on on left or right atrial catheterization
v wave on catheterization
v wave on pulmonary capillary wedge tracing
VA (ventriculoatrial) block cycle length
VA conduction
VA interval
VAD (ventricular assist device)
   Pierce-Donachy Thoratec
   Thoratec
vagal stimulation
Vairox high compression vascular stockings
Valsalva maneuver
valve (see also *prosthesis)*
   absent pulmonary
   Angell-Shiley bioprosthetic
   Angell-Shiley xenograft prosthetic
   Angiocor prosthetic
   annuloplasty
   aortic (AV)

valve *(cont.)*
   atrioventricular (AV)
   ball
   ball-and-cage prosthetic
   ball-cage
   Beall 106 prosthetic
   Beall-Surgitool 106 prosthetic
   Beall-Surgitool ball-cage prosthetic
   Beall-Surgitool disk prosthetic
   Beall-Surgitool prosthetic
   Bicer-val prosthetic
   bicuspid
   bicuspid aortic
   bicuspid pulmonary
   bi-leaflet tilting-disk prosthetic
   Biocor prosthetic
   bioprosthetic
   Bio-Vascular prosthetic
   Bjork-Shiley convexo-concave disk prosthetic
   Bjork-Shiley monostrut prosthetic
   Bjork-Shiley prosthetic aortic
   Bjork-Shiley prosthetic mitral
   bovine heart
   Braunwald-Cutter ball prosthetic
   butterfly heart
   C-C (convexo-concave) heart
   caged ball occluder prosthetic
   caged disk occluder prosthetic
   calcification of mitral
   calcified
   calcified aortic
   Capetown aortic prosthetic

valve *(cont.)*
Carpentier-Edwards aortic
Carpentier-Edwards bioprosthetic
Carpentier-Edwards mitral annuloplasty
Carpentier-Edwards pericardial
Carpentier-Edwards porcine prosthetic
Carpentier-Edwards Porcine SupraAnnular (SAV)
cleft mitral
commissural pulmonary
competent
congenital absence of pulmonary
congenital anomaly of mitral (CAMV)
congenital bicuspid aortic
congenital unicuspid
congenitally bicuspid aortic
congenitally quadricuspid aortic
convexo-concave disk prosthetic
Cooley-Cutter disk prosthetic
Coratomic prosthetic
Cross-Jones disk prosthetic
cryopreserved allograft heart
Cutter-Smeloff heart
DeBakey-Surgitool prosthetic
Delrin frame of
doming of
dysplastic
early opening of
eccentric monocuspid tilting-disk prosthetic
echo-dense
Edmark mitral
Edwards-Duromedics bi-leaflet
Edwards-Duromedics prosthetic
Elgiloy frame of prosthetic
eustachian
extirpation of
fibrotic mitral
flail mitral
floppy mitral
glutaraldehyde-tanned porcine heart

valve *(cont.)*
Gott shunt/butterfly heart
Guangzhou GD-1 prosthetic
Hall prosthetic heart
Hall-Kaster disk prosthetic
hammocking of
Hancock aortic 242 prosthetic
Hancock bioprosthetic
Hancock mitral 342 prosthetic
Hancock pericardial prosthetic
Hancock porcine heterograft
Hancock II porcine prosthetic
Hancock prosthetic mitral
Harken prosthetic
Hemex prosthetic
heterograft
hockey-stick tricuspid
Holter
Hufnagel prosthetic
hypoplastic
incompetent
Intact xenograft prosthetic
Ionescu-Shiley bioprosthetic
Ionescu-Shiley bovine pericardial
Ionescu-Shiley heart
Ionescu-Shiley low-profile prosthetic
Ionescu-Shiley standard pericardial prosthetic
Jatene-Macchi prosthetic
Kay-Shiley disk prosthetic
Kay-Shiley mitral
Kay-Suzuki disk prosthetic
leaky
Lillehei-Kaster disk prosthetic
Lillehei-Kaster pivoting-disk prosthetic
Lillehei-Kaster prosthetic mitral
Liotta-BioImplant LPB prosthetic
low-profile prosthetic
Magovern-Cromic ball prosthetic
Magovern-Cromic ball-cage prosthetic
Medtronic prosthetic
Medtronic-Hall heart

valve *(cont.)*
   Medtronic-Hall monocuspid tilting disk
   midsystolic buckling of mitral
   midsystolic closure of aortic
   mitral (MV)
   Mitroflow pericardial prosthetic
   narrowed
   native
   notching of pulmonic
   Omnicarbon prosthetic
   Omniscience prosthetic
   parachute mitral
   Pemco prosthetic
   porcine heart
   premature closure of
   premature mid-diastolic closure of mitral
   prosthetic
   Puig Massana-Shiley annuloplasty
   pulmonic; pulmonary (PV)
   quadricuspid pulmonary
   regurgitation of mitral
   rheumatic mitral
   semilunar
   Smeloff prosthetic
   Smeloff-Cutter ball prosthetic
   Smeloff-Cutter ball-cage prosthetic
   Sorin prosthetic
   Starr-Edwards prosthetic aortic
   Starr-Edwards prosthetic mitral
   Starr-Edwards Silastic
   Stellite ring material of prosthetic
   stenosis of mitral
   stenotic
   St. Jude bi-leaflet prosthetic
   St. Jude Medical bi-leaflet
   Surgitool 200 prosthetic
   systolic anterior motion of mitral
   Tascon prosthetic
   thickened mitral
   tilting-disk valve

valve *(cont.)*
   track
   tricuspid (TV)
   tricuspid aortic
   trileaflet aortic
   Ultracor prosthetic
   unicommissural aortic
   Vascor porcine prosthetic
   Wada-Cutter disk prosthetic
   Wessex prosthetic
   Xenomedica prosthetic
   Xenotech prosthetic
valve area
valve calcification
valve dehiscence
valve incompetence
valve of Vieussens
valve outflow strut
valve plane
valve replacement
valve tip
valvotomy
   aortic
   balloon
   double-balloon
   percutaneous mitral balloon (PMV)
   pulmonary
   single-balloon
valvular apparatus
valvular heart disease
valvular opening
valvular orifice
valvular regurgitation
valvulitis, rheumatic
valvuloplasty
   aortic
   bailout
   balloon
   balloon aortic
   balloon mitral
   balloon pulmonary (BPV)
   Carpentier tricuspid
   catheter balloon (CBV)
   double-balloon

valvuloplasty *(cont.)*
  Kay tricuspid
  percutaneous aortic (PAV)
  percutaneous balloon
  percutaneous balloon aortic
  percutaneous mitral balloon
    (PMV)
  pulmonary
  pulmonary balloon
  retrograde simultaneous double-balloon
  retrograde simultaneous single-balloon
  single-balloon
valvulotomy
valvulotome
  Gerbode mitral
  Himmelstein
  Leather venous
  Mills
valvulotomy
  open
  pulmonary
valvutome, Mills
Van Tassel pigtail catheter
variability, beat-to-beat
Variflex catheter
varicosity, varicosities
varix, varices
Vas recorder
Vas-Cath
vasa vasorum
Vascor porcine prosthetic valve
Vascoray contrast medium
vascular hemophilia
vascular tape
vasculature, pulmonary
vasculitis
  allergic
  hypersensitivity
  leukocytoclastic
  necrotizing
  nodular
  polyarteritis-like systemic
  segmented hyalinizing

vasculitis *(cont.)*
  toxic
vasoconstriction, peripheral
vasodepressor reaction (VDR)
vasodilate
vasodilator, peripheral
vasospastic angina
vasovagal episode
vasovagal orthostatism
vasovagal phenomenon
vasovagal syncope
VAT (ventricular activation time)
Vaughn Williams classification of antiarrhythmic drugs
VCB (ventricular capture beat)
V_{CF} (fiber-shortening velocity)
VCF (ventricular contractility function)
VD (valvular disease)
VDI (venous distensibility index)
VDR (vasodepressor reaction)
VEA (ventricular ectopic activity)
VEB (ventricular ectopic beat)
vector
  mean cardiac
  mean QRS
  P
  QRS
  ST
  T
  T wave
vector EKG
vector loop
vectorcardiogram, -graphy
  frontal plane
  sagittal plane
  transverse plane
Veg. (vegetation)
vegetation, valvular
vein, veins
  autogenous
  Boyd perforating
  distended neck
  distention of neck
  Dodd perforating group of

vein *(cont.)*
  flat neck
  Marshall
  thebesian
  varicose
vein harvesting
vein stripping operation
velocimetry, Doppler
velocity
  coronary blood flow (CBFV)
  diastolic regurgitant
  fiber-shortening (V$_{CF}$)
  maximal transaortic jet
  mean aortic flow
  mean posterior wall
  mean pulmonary flow
  meter per second (m/sec)
  peak aortic flow
  peak flow
  peak pulmonary flow
  peak transmitted
  regurgitant
vena cava (pl., venae cavae)
  inferior (IVC)
  superior (SVC)
VenES II Medical Stockings
Venflon cannula
venipuncture
venoarterial admixture
venogram, venography
  isotope
  radionuclide
  technetium-99m
venostasis
venotomy
venous access
venous cannula
venous cutdown
venous distention
venous Doppler exam
venous hum (nun's murmur)
venous reservoir
venous stasis
venous ulcer

vent
  intracardiac
  pulmonary arterial
  slotted needle
Ventak AICD (automatic implantable cardioverter-defibrillator) pacemaker
venting
ventilation
  intermittent mandatory (IMV)
  mechanical
  pressure-cycled
  synchronized intermittent mandatory (SIMV)
  time-cycled
  volume-cycled
ventilator, MA-1
ventilator/resuscitator, pneuPAC
venting aortic Bengash-type needle
ventricle
  akinetic left
  atrialized
  auxillary
  common
  double-inlet
  double-outlet
  double-outlet right (DORV)
  dysfunctional left
  hypokinetic left
  hypoplastic
  left (LV)
  Mary Allen Engle
  right (RV)
  rudimentary right
  single
Ventricor pacemaker
ventricular activation time (VAT)
ventricular aneurysm
ventricular apex
ventricular capture beat
ventricular cavity
ventricular contraction pattern
ventricular dysfunction
ventricular ectopy

ventricular effective refractory
 period (VERP)
ventricular elastance, maximum
 (E$_{MAX}$)
ventricular enlargement
ventricular extrastimulation
ventricular fibrillation
ventricular function curve
ventricular hypertrophy
ventricular lead
ventricular overdrive pacing
ventricular paroxysmal tachycardia
ventricular preexcitation
ventricular premature contraction
ventricular premature depolarization
 (VPD)
ventricular pressure, right
ventricular rate
ventricular refractoriness
ventricular refractory period
ventricular response
 fast
 moderate
 rapid
 slow
ventricular rhythm disturbance
ventricular segmental contraction
ventricular septal defect (VSD)
ventricular septal rupture
ventricular septal summit
ventricular single and double
 extrastimulation
ventricular systole
ventricular tachycardia (VT), recurrent intractable
ventricular wall motion
ventricularization of left atrial
 pressure pulse
ventricularized morphology
ventriculoarterial conduit
ventriculoatrial effective refractory
 period
ventriculoatrial time-out
ventriculogram, -graphy
 axial left anterior oblique

ventriculogram *(cont.)*
 biplane
 digital subtraction
 dipyridamole thallium
 exercise radionuclide
 first-pass radionuclide
 gated blood pool
 gated nuclear
 gated radionuclide
 LAO (left anterior oblique)
  projection
 left (LVG)
 radionuclide (RNV)
 RAO (right anterior oblique)
  projection
 retrograde left
 single plane left
 xenon^{133}
ventriculorrhaphy
 linear
 Reed
ventriculotomy
 encircling endocardial
 endocardial
 transmural
ventriculo-arterial discordance
venule
VeriFlex guide wire
VERP (ventricular effective refractory period)
verrucous carditis
Versatrax pacemaker
Versatrax II pacemaker
Versatrax pulse generator
vertebral-basilar arterial insufficiency
vertebrobasilar insufficiency
vessel, vessels
 atherectomized
 caliber of
 codominant
 collateral
 contralateral
 cross-pelvic collateral
 dominant

vessel *(cont.)*
  great
  nondominant
  patent
  peripelvic collateral
vessel loop
Vesseloops rubber band
VF (ventricular fibrillation)
VFT (venous filling time)
VH interval
viability, tissue
Viagraph computerized exercise EKG system
Vicor pacemaker
Vicryl suture
videoangiography, digital
Vieussens
  circle of
  valve of
view
  anterior
  apical four-chamber (echocardiogram)
  caudal
  four-chamber apical
  ice-pick M-mode echocardiogram
  LAO (left anterior oblique)
  LAO-cranial
  left anterior oblique (LAO)
  long-axis parasternal
  parasternal long-axis echocardiogram
  parasternal short-axis
  RAO (right anterior oblique)
  RAO-caudal
  right anterior oblique (RAO)
  short-axis parasternal
  sitting-up
  spider x-ray
  subcostal four-chamber echocardiogram
  subcostal long-axis echocardiogram
  subcostal short-axis echocardiogram

view *(cont.)*
  subxiphoid echocardiography
  suprasternal notch (echocardiogram)
  weeping willow x-ray
Vigilon dressing
Vineberg cardiac revascularization procedure
VingMed ultrasound
visceral heterotaxy
visceral pericardium
viscosity
  blood
  plasma
Vista pacemaker
Vital Cooley microvascular needleholder
Vital Ryder microvascular needleholder
Vitalcor venous catheter
Vitamin K
Vitatrax pacemaker
Vitatron catheter electrode
Vitatron pacemaker
VLDL (very-low-density lipoprotein)
VLDL-TG (VLDL-triglyceride)
VLDL-TG/HDL-C ratio
VLP (ventricular late potential)
VO_2 (ventilatory oxygen consumption)
Volkmann retractor
volt
voltage
  battery
  increased (on EKG)
  low
  precordial
voltage criteria
volume
  atrial emptying
  blood
  cavity
  chamber
  circulation
  diastolic atrial

volume (cont.)
   Dodge area-length method for ventricular
   endocardial
   end-diastolic
   end-systolic (ESV)
   end-systolic residual
   epicardial
   forward stroke (FSV)
   left ventricular chamber
   left ventricular end-diastolic
   left ventricular inflow (LVIV)
   left ventricular outflow (LVOV)
   left ventricular stroke
   LV (left ventricular) cavity
   mean corpuscular (MCV)
   minute
   plasma
   prism method for ventricular
   pulmonary blood
   pyramid method for ventricular
   radionuclide stroke
   regurgitant stroke (RSV)
   right ventricular
   Simpson rule method for ventricular
   stroke (SV)
   systolic atrial
   Teichholz equation for left ventricular

volume (cont.)
   thermodilution stroke
   total stroke (TSV)
   ventricular end-diastolic
   von Recklinghausen test
volume depletion, intravascular
volume infusion
volume overload
von Willebrand blood coagulation factor
von Willebrand disease; syndrome
VOO pacemaker
Vorse-Webster clamp
VPB (ventricular premature beat)
VPC (ventricular premature complex; contraction)
VPD (ventricular premature depolarization)
VPT (ventricular paroxysmal tachycardia)
VRT (venous return time)
VSD (ventricular septal defect) (see *defect*)
VT (ventricular tachycardia)
VT/VF (ventricular tachycardia/ventricular fibrillation)
VVI pacemaker
VVI/AAI pacemaker
VVT pacemaker

W

W pattern on right atrial waveform
W wave on echocardiogram
Waardenburg syndrome
Wada-Cutter disk prosthetic valve
waist, cardiac
waist of balloon catheter
Waldhausen subclavian flap technique

wall
   akinetic
   aneurysmal
   anterior
   anterior chest
   anterior left ventricular
   anterobasal
   anterolateral

wall *(cont.)*
   anterolateral ventricular
   aortic
   apical
   atrial free
   basal
   chest
   diaphragmatic
   dilatation of ventricular free
   friable
   inferior
   inferior left ventricular
   inferoposterior
   lateral
   left ventricular free (LVFW)
   left ventricular posterior (LVPW)
   midventricular
   myocardial
   posterior left ventricular
   posterolateral ventricular
   posterior (PW)
   posterobasal
   posterobasilar
   posterolateral
   right ventricular free (RVFW)
   septal
   thickening of ventricular
   vessel
wall motion (see *motion)*
wall motion abnormality (see *abnormality)*
wall motion score
wall motion score index
wall motion study
wall sluggishness
wall thickening
wall thickness
wall thinning
wandering atrial pacemaker (WAP)
wandering baseline
Wangensteen anastomosis clamp
Wangensteen patent ductus clamp
WAP (wandering atrial pacemaker)
Ward-Romano syndrome

Wardrop method
washer, felt
washout, delayed
washout rate
water brash (heartburn)
water-hammer pulse
water seal, chest tube to
Waterston extrapericardial anastomosis
Waterston groove
Waterston pacing wire
Waterston shunt
Waterston-Cooley shunt
watt-seconds
wave
   A (cardiac apex pulse; right atrial pressure)
   "a" (jugular venous pulse)
   anacrotic
   atrial repolarization
   bifid P
   biphasic P
   biphasic T
   C
   c (jugular venous pulse)
   Cannon "a" (jugular venous pulse)
   CV
   cv (jugular venous pulse)
   D
   deep S
   delta
   dicrotic
   diphasic P
   diphasic T
   dysphasic
   echocardiogram "a"
   enlarged T
   f (jugular venous pulse)
   flat P
   flat T
   flattening of T
   flipped T
   flutter
   giant "a" (jugular venous pulse)

wave *(cont.)*
  h (jugular venous pulse)
  hyperacute T
  inverted P
  inverted Q
  inverted T
  inverted U
  inversion of T
  J
  low-amplitude
  nonconducted P
  nondiagnostic Q
  non-Q
  nonspecific T
  notched P
  Osborn
  P
  pathologic Q
  peaked P
  percussion
  pointed P
  postexcitation
  pulse
  Q
  QRS
  QS
  R
  r (jugular venous pulse)
  rapid filling (RFW)
  RF (cardiac apex pulse)
  R' (R prime)
  R'R"
  S
  septal Q
  SF (cardiac apex pulse)
  sharp
  ST
  T
  Ta
  T upright
  tall P
  tall R
  terminal negativity of P
  tidal
  TU

wave *(cont.)*
  U
  upright R
  upright T
  upright U
  V (right atrial pressure)
  v (jugular venous pulse)
  v (pulmonary capillary wedge tracing)
  W
  widened P
  x' (right atrial catheterization)
  x descent of the "a"
  y descent of the "a"
wave amplitude
waveform, pressure
waveform analysis
waveform from arterial line
wave inversion
wax, bone
waxing and waning in intensity
WBC (white blood cell) count, *consisting of:*
  bands (immature neutrophils)
  basos (basophils)
  blasts
  eos (eosinophils)
  lymphs (lymphocytes)
  monos (monocytes)
  neutrophils
  polys or PMNs (polymorphonuclear leukocytes)
  segs (segmented neutrophils)
WBC with differential (diff)
weaned off cardiopulmonary bypass
weaned from respirator; ventilator
Webb vein stripper
Weber aortic clamp
Webster coronary sinus catheter
Webster infusion cannula
web, inferior vena cava
Weck clip; clipped
wedge position
weeping willow x-ray view
Weinberg rib spreader

Weitlaner retractor
well, pericardial
Wenck. Phen. (Wenckebach phenomenon)
Wenckebach block
Wenckebach cardioptosis
Wenckebach cycle
Wenckebach disease
Wenckebach pathway
Wenckebach period
Wenckebach phenomenon
Wessex prosthetic valve
Westergren method
Westergren sedimentation rate
Westphal forceps
wheal, skin
whiff of dye
Wholey Hi-Torque Floppy guide wire
Wholey Hi-Torque Modified J guide wire
Wholey Hi-Torque Standard guide wire
Wholey wire
whorling of myocardial cells
wide complex rhythm
widely split second sound
widened cardiac silhouette
Wigle scale for ventricular hypertrophy
Willauer thoracic scissors
Williams L-R guiding catheter
Williams syndrome
Wilmer scissors
Wilson central terminal on EKG lead
Wilson rib spreader
Wilton-Webster catheter
wind sock sign on echocardiogram
window
    acoustic
    aortic
    aorticopulmonary
    aortopulmonary
Winiwarter-Buerger disease
wire, wires
    Amplatz torque
    atrial pacing
    Bentson
    coronary
    dock; docking
    epicardial pacing
    flexible steerable
    floppy tipped guide
    guide (see *guide wire*)
    J tip
    J tipped guide
    Killip
    pacing (see *electrode*)
    steerable
    sternal
    Stertzer-Myler extension
    temporary pacing
    Waterston pacing
    Wholey
wire cutter
wiry pulse
withdrawn
Wister vascular clamp
within normal limits (WNL)
Wizard disposable inflation device
WNL (within normal limits)
Wolff-Parkinson-White (WPW) syndrome
Wolvek sternal approximator
Wood units index for resistance
Woodward hemostat
work
    left ventricular stroke (LVSW)
    right ventricular stroke (RVSW)
workload of heart
    5-MET
    7-MET
    Bruce stage
    increased
wound, separate stab
woven graft
wrapping of abdominal aortic aneurysm
Wylie carotid artery clamp

X

x depression of jugular venous
  pulse
x descent of the "a" wave
x descent of jugular venous pulse
x' (x prime) wave pressure on right
  atrial catheterization
xanthelasma
xanthoma
  eruptive
  palmar
  tendinous
  tuberoeruptive
  tuberous

xenograft (heterograft) (see *graft)*
Xenomedica prosthetic valve
xenon-133 ventriculography
Xenotech prosthetic valve
xiphisternal region
xiphoid area; process
x-ray
  baseline chest
  chest (CXR)
Xyrel pacemaker
XYZ lead system, Frank EKG

Y

Y connector, ACS angioplasty
y depression of jugular venous
  pulse
y descent of the "a" wave
y descent of jugular venous pulse
Y-shaped graft

y wave pressure on right atrial
  catheterization
Yankauer suction tube
Yasargil artery forceps
Yasargil carotid clamp

Z

Z point
z point pressure on left atrial
  catheterization
z point pressure on right atrial
  catheterization
Zener diode
Zimmer antiembolism support
  stockings
zipper scar
Zitron pacemaker

ZK44012 contrast medium
Zoll NTP noninvasive temporary
  pacemaker
zone
  ischemic
  transition
ZSC (zone of slow conduction)
Zucker #7 French catheter
Zwenger test

References

References

Cardiology

ACTA Cardiologica: International Journal of Cardiology, 43:2 (1988).

American Heart Journal, 116:4 (Oct 1988); 117:1 (Jan 1989); 117:2 (Feb 1989); 117:3 (Mar 1989). St. Louis: C. V. Mosby Co.

American Journal of Cardiology, 62:15 (11 Nov 1988); 63:1 (1 Jan 1989); 63:3 (15 Jan 1989); 63:5 (1 Feb 1989); 63:7 (15 Feb 1989); 63:8 (21 Feb); 63:9 (1 Mar 1989); 63:10 (7 Mar 1989); 63:11 (15 Mar 1989). Denver: Yorke Medical Journal, Cahners Publishing Co.

Andreoli, Kathleen G. DSN, et al. *Comprehensive Cardiac Care,* 6th ed. St. Louis: C. V. Mosby Co., 1987.

Angiology: The Journal of Vascular Diseases, 40:1 (Jan 1989). New York: Westminster Publications, Inc.

Brandenburg, Robert O., M.D., et al. *Cardiology: Fundamentals and Practice.* Chicago: Year Book Medical Publishers, Inc., 1987.

Cheng, Tsung O., M.D. *The International Textbook of Cardiology.* New York: Pergamon Press, 1986.

Circulation, 79:1 (Jan 1989); 79:2 (Feb 1989); 79:3 (Mar 1989). Dallas: American Heart Association.

Clinical Cardiology: A Journal for Advances in Cardiovascular Disease, Vol. 12 (Mar 1989). Mahwah, N.J.: Foundation for Advances in Clinical Medicine, Inc.

Iskandrian, Abdulmassih S., M.D. *Nuclear Cardiac Imaging: Principles and Applications.* Philadelphia: F. A. Davis Co., 1987.

Journal of the American College of Cardiology, 13:2 (Feb 1989); 13:1 (Jan 1989); 13:3 (1 Mar 1989); 13:4 (15 Mar 1989).

Journal of Cardiovascular Surgery, 29:1 (Jan-Feb 1988); 29:6 (Nov-Dec 1988). Turin, Italy: Minerva Medica.

PACE: Pacing and Clinical Electrophysiology, 12:4 (Apr 1989). Mt. Kisco, NY: Futura Publishing Co., Inc.

Pohost, Gerald M., M.D., et al. *New Concepts in Cardiac Imaging, 1988.* Chicago: Year Book Medical Publishers, Inc., 1988.

Progress in Cardiovascular Diseases, 30:5 (Mar/Apr 1988); 30:6 (May/Jun 1988); 31:3 (Nov/Dec 1988); 31:4 (Jan/Feb 1989). Philadelphia: Grune & Stratton, Harcourt Brace Jovanovich, Inc.

The SUM Program Cardiology Transcription Unit. Modesto, Ca.: Health Professions Institute, 1989.

Surgical Clinics of North America, Latest Advances in Cardiac Surgery, 65:3 (Jun 1985); *Vascular Surgery,* 66:2 (Apr 1986); *Cardiothoracic Surgery,* 68:3 (Jun 1988). Philadelphia: W. B. Saunders Co.

Yan, Sing San, M.D., et al. *From Cardiac Catheterization Data to Hemodynamic Parameters.* Philadelphia: F. A. Davis Co., 1988.

Yu, Paul N., M.D., and John F. Goodwin, M.D. *Progress in Cardiology.* Vols. 15, 16. Philadelphia: Lea & Febiger, 1987, 1988.

General Medicine and Surgery

Bennington, James L., M.D. *Saunders Dictionary & Encyclopedia of Laboratory Medicine and Technology.* Philadelphia: W. B. Saunders Co., 1984.

Billups, Norman F., and Shirley M. Billups. *American Drug Index.* 33rd ed. Philadelphia: J. B. Lippincott Co., 1989.

Campbell, Linda C. *The Anatomy Word Book.* Modesto, Ca.: Prima Vera Publications, 1989.

Crowley, Leonard V., M.D. *Introduction to Human Diseases.* 2nd ed. Boston: Jones and Bartlett, 1988.

Dirckx, John H., M.D. *H & P: A Nonphysician's Guide to the Medical History and Physical Examination.* Modesto, Ca.: Prima Vera Publications, 1987.

Dorland's Illustrated Medical Dictionary. 27th ed. Philadelphia: W. B. Saunders Co., 1988.

Drug Facts and Comparisons. St. Louis: J. B. Lippincott Co., 1989.

Fuller, Joanna R. *Surgical Technology: Principles and Practice.* 2nd ed. Philadelphia: W. B. Saunders Co., 1986.

Gruendemann, Barbara J., and Margaret H. Meeker. *Alexander's Care of the Patient in Surgery.* 8th ed. St. Louis: C. V. Mosby Co., 1987.

Logan, Carolynn M., and M. Katherine Rice. *Logan's Medical and Scientific Abbreviations.* Philadelphia: J. B. Lippincott Co., 1987.

Melloni's Illustrated Medical Dictionary. 2nd ed. Ed. by Dox, Melloni, and Eisner. Baltimore: Williams & Wilkins Publishing Co., 1985.

The Merck Manual. 15th ed. Rahway, N.J.: Merck & Co., 1987.

Miller, Benjamin F., and Claire Brackman Keane. *Encyclopedia and Dictionary of Medicine, Nursing, and Allied Health.* 4th ed. Philadelphia: W. B. Saunders, 1987.

Physicians' Desk Reference. 43rd ed. Oradell, N.J.: Medical Economics Co., 1989.

Physicians' Desk Reference for Nonprescription Drugs. 10th ed. Oradell, N.J.: Medical Economics Co., 1989.

Pyle, Vera. *Current Medical Terminology.* 2nd ed. Modesto, Ca.: Prima Vera Publications, 1988.

Roe-Hafer, Ann. *The Medical & Health Sciences Word Book*. 2nd ed. Boston: Houghton Mifflin Co., 1982.

Smith, F. J. and Y. R. *Smiths' Reference and Illustrated Guide to Surgical Instruments*. Philadelphia: J. B. Lippincott Co., 1983.

Stedman's Medical Dictionary. 24th ed. Baltimore: Williams & Wilkins Co., 1982.

Taber's Cyclopedic Medical Dictionary. 16th ed. Ed. by Clayton L. Thomas. Philadelphia: F. A. Davis Co., 1989.

Tighe, Shirley M. Brooks. *Instrumentation for the Operating Room: A Photographic Manual*. 3rd ed. St. Louis: C. V. Mosby Co., 1989.

Webster's Medical Desk Dictionary. Springfield, Mass.: Merriam-Webster, Inc., Publishers, 1986.

Style, Grammar, Mechanics

Chicago Manual of Style. 13th ed. Chicago: The University of Chicago Press, 1982.

Diehl, Marcy O., and Marilyn T. Fordney. *Medical Typing and Transcribing: Techniques and Procedures*. 2nd ed. Philadelphia: W. B. Saunders Co., 1984.

Dirckx, John H., M.D. *The Language of Medicine: Its Evolution, Structure, and Dynamics*. 2nd ed. New York: Praeger Publishers, 1983.

Fowler, H. W. *A Dictionary of Modern English Usage*. 2nd ed. Rev. by Sir Ernest Gowers. New York: Oxford University Press, 1985.

Johnson, Edward D. *The Handbook of Good English*. New York: Facts on File Publications, 1982.

Manual for Authors & Editors: Editorial Style & Manuscript Preparation. 7th ed. Compiled for American Medical Association by William R. Barclay et al. Los Altos, Ca.: Lange Medical Publications, 1981.

Shertzer, Margaret. *The Elements of Grammar*. New York: Macmillan Publishing Co., 1986.

Tessier, Claudia, and Sally C. Pitman. *Style Guide for Medical Transcription*. Modesto, Ca.: American Association for Medical Transcription, 1985.

Webster's Standard American Style Manual. Springfield, Mass.: Merriam-Webster, Inc., Publishers, 1985.

Words into Type. Based on studies by Marjorie E. Skillin et al. 3rd ed. Englewood Cliffs, N.J.: Prentice-Hall, Inc., 1974.

English Dictionaries

The American Heritage Dictionary. 2nd ed. New York: Houghton Mifflin Co., 1983.

The New Lexicon Webster's Dictionary of the English Language. New York: Lexicon Publications, Inc., 1987.

Oxford American Dictionary. Compiled by Eugene Ehrlich et al. New York: Oxford University Press, 1980.

The Random House Dictionary of the English Language. 2nd ed., Unabridged. Ed. by Flexner and Hauck. New York: Random House, 1987.

Webster's Ninth New Collegiate Dictionary. Springfield, Mass.: Merriam-Webster, Inc., Publishers, 1983.